Swine Practice

The *In Practice* Handbooks Series

Series Editor: Edward Boden

Past and present members of *In Practice* Editorial Board

Titles in print:
Feline Practice
Canine Practice
Equine Practice
Bovine Practice
Sheep and Goat Practice
Swine Practice

The *In Practice* Handbooks

Swine Practice

Edited by E. Boden
Executive Editor, *In Practice*

Baillière Tindall

LONDON   PHILADELPHIA   TORONTO   SYDNEY   TOKYO

Baillière Tindall   24–28 Oval Road
W. B. Saunders   London NW1 7DX

The Curtis Center
Independence Square West
Philadelphia, PA 19106–3399, USA

55 Horner Avenue
Toronto, Ontario, M8Z 4X6, Canada

Harcourt Brace Jovanovich Group
(Australia) Pty Ltd
30–52 Smidmore Street
Marrickville
NSW 2204, Australia

Harcourt Brace Jovanovich Japan Inc
Ichibancho Central Building
22–1 Ichibancho
Chiyoda-ku, Tokyo 102, Japan

Typeset by Photo·graphics, Honiton, Devon
Printed and bound in Hong Kong by Dah Hua Printing
Press Co., Ltd.

A catalogue record for this book is available from
the British Library

ISBN 0–7020–1557–1

Contents

CONTROL

Contributors

T. J. L. Alexander Deputy Head, Department of Clinical Veterinary Medicine, University of Cambridge, Madingley Road, Cambridge CB3 0ES, UK

J. Carr Lecturer in Pig Health and Productivity, Department of Animal Health, Royal Veterinary College, University of London, Boltons Park, Hawkshead Road, Potters Bar, Hertfordshire EN6 1NB, UK

F. Clifton-Hadley *Formerly* Research Associate, University of Cambridge, Cambridge, UK

R. G. A. Douglas Douglas and MacKinnon Veterinary Surgeons, Station Road, Framlingham, Woodbridge, Suffolk IP13 9EE, UK

C. Glossop Research Officer, Reading Cattle Breeding Centre, Shinfield, Nr Reading, Berkshire, UK

T. W. Heard Grove House, Corston, Malmesbury, Wiltshire SN16 0HL, UK

M. Meredith Lecturer in Clinical Veterinary Medicine, Animal Health Division, University of Cambridge, Department of Clinical Veterinary Medicine, Madingley Road, Cambridge CB3 0ES, UK

W. M. Miller Pig Improvement Company Inc., PO Box 348, Franklin, Kentucky 4213, USA

J. Oldham Veterinary Adviser, Cotswold Pig Development Co. Ltd, Rothwell, Lincoln L64 7TE, UK

W. J. Smith Senior Veterinary Information Officer, Scottish Agricultural Colleges, Veterinary Information Service, Mill of

Craibstone, Bucksburn, Aberdeen AB2 9BS, UK

D. Taylor   Senior Lecturer, Department of Veterinary Pathology, University of Glasgow, Bearsden Road, Bearsden, Glasgow G61 1QH, UK

J. Walton   Senior Lecturer, Farm Animal Division, University of Liverpool, Veterinary Field Station, Leahurst, Neston, Wirral, Merseyside L64 7TE, UK

G. A. H. Wells   Senior Research Officer, Ministry of Agriculture, Research Service, Department of Pathology, Central Veterinary Laboratory, New Haw, Weybridge, Surrey KT15 3NB, UK

M. E. C. White   Veterinary Surgeon, Haven Veterinary Group, 34 Ketwell Lane, Hedon, Hull, HU12 8BP, UK

Foreword

In Practice was started in 1979 as a clinical supplement to *The Veterinary Record*. Its carefully chosen, highly illustrated articles specially commissioned from leaders in their field were aimed specifically at the practitioner. They have proved extremely popular with experienced veterinarians and students alike. The editorial board, chaired for the first 10 years by Professor James Armour, was particularly concerned to emphasize differential diagnosis.

In response to consistent demand, articles from *In Practice*, updated and revised by the authors, are now published in convenient handbook form. Each book deals with a particular species or group of related animals.

E. Boden

Production

CHAPTER 1

Pig Recording for Production and Profit

JOHN OLDHAM

INTRODUCTION

Since the late 1960s tremendous progress has been made in convincing pig producers of the need for good recording practice. It is probably true to say that those who remain unconvinced are no longer in pig business anyway!

The first essential of any recording system is *standard definitions* of all parameters used. Surprisingly, standardization is of more importance than strict accuracy, in order that valid comparisons may be made between different herds, different systems and even different countries. The difficulty of achieving absolute accuracy may be illustrated by the UK standard definition of "stillborn piglets" from *Pig Health Recording, Production and Finance – A Producers Guide*; produced in association with the Pig Veterinary Society (1986): "Piglets found dead behind the sow after farrowing. Note: If necessary, confirmed by post mortem examination to determine if the piglets have breathed".

Clearly it is unreasonable to expect a pigman to open every suspected piglet to determine if it has breathed, but should the standard definition reveal the need for investigation, a series of post-mortem examinations would be useful in assessing the true extent of the problem.

Table 1.1 Recording methods

Individual animal	e.g. sow, boar
Herd	e.g. breeding, feeding
Production	e.g. day-to-day management, period management
Financial	e.g. period costings, period accounting
Analytical	problem identification, problem solving
Manual/computerized	

There are many ways of categorizing records. The list in Table 1.1 is not intended to be complete but will perhaps provide a basis for more detailed examination.

CHOOSING YOUR RECORDING METHOD

There are clearly all manner of combinations between the different methods in Table 1.1, and individual requirements have to be taken into account before a decision on "system" is taken.

Given the sophistication of present-day pig production some requirements seem to be essential in order to arrive at good production and financial decisions, and also to offer data-processing facilities for advisers, especially veterinarians. The ability to analyse data successfully, perhaps over long or comparable periods, is clearly very important, and the author would submit that, as one can never be sure in advance which parameters will be required for analysis, a *fully interactive data base management system (computerized)* is likely to be the only really satisfactory answer.

COMPUTERIZED SYSTEMS

Computer based systems may be "on-farm", or "bureau" usually using postal communications. For such systems to be fully satisfactory the "turnaround" period must not be more than 3 days and on a weekly basis, if the system is intended for day-to-day production management. On-farm systems (Fig. 1.1) may be less powerful than bureau systems and require great discipline to ensure regular data inputs, error checking, etc. Prerequisites of any computerized system include standardized coding, and a simple "idiot-proof" method of data collection without duplication or subsequent form filling. Routine output should be restricted to useful information only, with minimum use of confusing numbers and maximum use of graphics.

DATA COLLECTION

Reporting by exception is a good technique, e.g. reporting abortions only when their numbers exceed an agreed interference level. As previously stated there must be a powerful analytical capability to include all data entered.

Individual sow (and boar) information must be the source from which all analyses are derived, thus allowing rational decisions, for instance on culling, to be made regarding individual animals in the breeding herd.

Key production parameters in the breeding herd are normally measured against agreed targets. They would include:

Sow herd size (average over 12 months).
Farrowing rate – "The number of sows which farrow to a given number of services expressed as a percentage".
Farrowing index – "The number of farrowings taking place in an agreed period divided by the average number of sows in the herd and grossed up or down to a 365-day period".
Litter size – "The total number of piglets born per litter, including still-born and mummified". Can also be expressed separately as live, stillborn, or mummified piglets per litter.
Weaning (piglets) – "The act of permanently removing piglets from the sow". Recording the details of each weaning produces the figure "pigs weaned per litter".
Pigs born, weaned, and sold per sow per year are also important measures of production.

These parameters form an important part of the management period production records, rather than "day-to-day" (or "week-by-week"), which are so important in achieving regular and satisfactory results. The figure shows a "services cu-sum" designed to keep the stockman constantly aware of performance against a target-line on a cumulative basis.

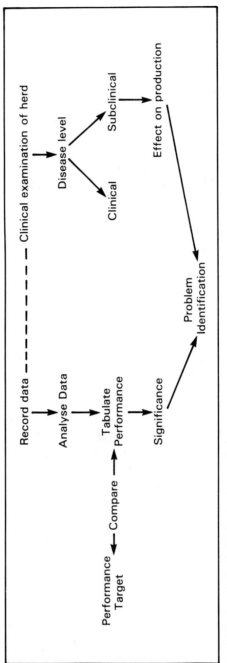

Fig. 1.1 A pathway for the identification of problems on the farm.

THE FEEDING HERD

The feeding herd requires a rather different approach to recording, and the importance of this area is only exceeded by its neglect. In 1986, BOCM Silcock, following a large-scale survey, found that "one third of fattening herds don't bother to record at all and many of those which do fail to weigh their pigs". When one considers that an increase in feed conversion of 0.1 in the UK costs about £1, it is ludicrous that farmers should say that "recording was too complicated, took up too much time, and was too expensive". In practice on-farm growth trial work can be shown to be highly cost effective and great savings can be made provided that significant numbers can be included in each trial group. Essential parameters in the feeding herd include daily liveweight gain, feed conversion efficiency and cost per lb (or kg) liveweight (or deadweight).

Most recording systems are able to produce these figures for a whole herd over long periods without accurate weighings, on the basis of opening and closing stock estimates. However such information is historical, and of no help in highlighting current problems. Figures 1.2 and 1.3 and Table 1.2 (standard output from "Pigtales" recording system) show how computer output, perhaps coupled with actual weighings, can constantly monitor growth rates, the "lot number" approach being particularly useful as an "early warning system". "Lots" need to be identified with their pens, and immaculate records of movement between "lots" must be kept. The computer automatically corrects for age in the case of recorded movements.

It is also possible to run such a system on a manual rather than computerized basis.

FINANCIAL RECORDS

Financial records are rarely of use on a short-term basis, and financial accounts are most useful for assessing "bottom line" profitability after interest and other financial charges, partly to confirm solvency, and partly to determine tax liability! Financial costings on the other hand can be used against targets (or budget), and from the adviser's point of view a

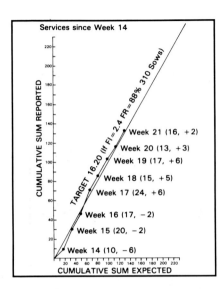

Fig. 1.2
Breeder service recording system output for client's farm May 1988, showing cumulative sum performance against target for services since week 14 (Pigtales Recording System).

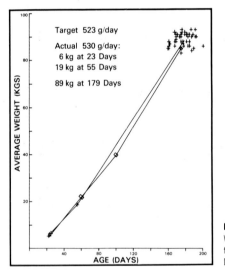

Fig. 1.3
Weight for age performance against age for client farm. Lots weighed 1 October 1987 to 31 December 1987 (Pigtales Recording System).

rough but very useful guide to profitability in the herd is the cost of feed as a percentage of total sales.

Indeed, this same approach can be used very effectively to measure efficiency in other areas provided the "norms" for the industry are known. Labour, electricity, veterinary costs,

Table 1.2 Current lots report from client's farm, May 1988 (Pigtales Recording System).

Lot	Started	Start	Transfers		Losses	Selected	Sold	Remaining	Age
1	10.12.87	143+	0+	0–	0–	0–	133–	10	194*
2	18.12.87	120+	0+	0–	2–	0–	82–	36	185*
3	24.12.87	122+	0+	6–	10–	5–	54–	47	178*
4	30.12.87	118+	0+	0–	5–	3–	13–	97	172
5	8. 1.88	62+	62+	1–	0–	3–	4–	116	163
6	15. 1.88	136+	30+	60–	1–	0–	0–	105	158
7	22. 1.88	139+	5+	39–	3–	0–	0–	102	153
8	29. 1.88	122+	6+	0–	5–	0–	0–	123	143
9	5. 2.88	147+	6+	0–	1–	0–	1–	151	137
10	12. 2.88	121+	0+	10–	2–	0–	0–	109	129
11	19. 2.88	74+	45+	1–	6–	0–	0–	112	120
12	26. 2.88	146+	12+	48–	2–	0–	0–	108	116
13	4. 3.88	115+	35+	4–	1–	0–	33–	112	107
14	11. 3.88	180+	0+	30–	4–	0–	27–	119	101
15	18. 3.88	159+	1+	0–	3–	0–	0–	157	94
16	25. 3.88	139+	56+	1–	2–	0–	0–	192	86
17	29. 3.88	131+	90+	56–	3–	0–	0–	162	79
18	8. 4.88	193+	0+	116–	0–	0–	0–	77	74
19	15. 4.88	167+	27+	4–	7–	0–	0–	183	67
20	22. 4.88	141+	4+	0–	9–	0–	0–	136	59
21	29. 4.88	112+	0+	0–	3–	0–	0–	109	52
22	6. 5.88	146+	0+	0–	0–	0–	0–	146	46
23	13. 5.88	177+	0+	60–	0–	0–	0–	117	37
24	19. 5.88	129+	30+	0–	3–	0–	0–	156	33
25	26. 5.88	94+	30+	0–	0–	0–	0–	124	28

*Indicates lots over 175 days old.

and many others can usefully be included, and this method often points the way towards the identification of areas of production inefficiencies.

WHOLE HERD VERSUS INDIVIDUAL RECORDS

The pathway for identifying problems already referred to shows clearly how data analysis can be used in conjunction with clinical examination to help identify and therefore correct a problem. The same pathway is often of value in looking at problems with individual animals, e.g. do we treat or cull?

On a whole herd (enterprise) basis, it is easy to identify an unsatisfactory farrowing index relative to target and actual weaning age. It is a different matter identifying the underlying causes, and ready access to *all* the relevant data is vital.

It is obvious that any veterinary adviser investigating poor reproductive performance needs a powerful analytical tool in order to be able to identify and correct the shortfall in production. Such analyses frequently highlight the multifactorial or multifaceted nature of so many problems in the modern intensive pig herd. Powerful analytical abilities also frequently show that the stockman's perception of the nature of the problem does not accord with the demonstrable facts.

"Whole-herd" or "enterprise" analysis is limited in the useful information it can provide; usually only averages and trends. Individual animal records allow a much more informative overview of distribution. Coupled with the use of histograms this becomes a powerful aid to problem-solving, as well as allowing all concerned to keep an eye on trends

Table 1.3 Factors which may influence farrowing index

Weaning to effective service interval
Returns to service (regular and irregular)
Abortions
Farrowing rate
Gestation length
Failure to farrow
Failure to detect returns
Failure to cull immediately decision is made

such as parity distribution within the herd, correct boar work levels, farrowing rate, and many others.

MOTIVATION

Finally a word on motivation. It is frequently difficult to convince stockpersons of the value of record keeping, especially as it may be seen as a tool for criticism by management. If on the other hand improvements in performance can be shown categorically by the recording system to follow the carrying out of specific advice, then there automatically follows an improvement in attitude towards the adviser, and a justified improvement in the stockperson's own self-esteem!

ACKNOWLEDGEMENT

Thanks to Pigtales Recording Systems.

REFERENCES AND FURTHER READING

Pig Health. Recording, Production and Finance. A Producer's Guide. Produced in association with the Pig Veterinary Society, c/o BVA, 7 Mansfield St, London W1M 0AT.
Fatteners thin on recording. *Pig Farming Magazine*, Dec, 1986.

CHAPTER 2

Poor Production in Growing Pigs

JOHN WALTON

INTRODUCTION

Over the past decade there has been a conscious effort to keep staffing levels as low as possible on all pig units. Although on paper this has been attractive from an accounting point of view, the effect on pig health, welfare and productivity has, in many cases, been counterproductive. Certain areas of the production cycle require minimal attention from the stockman but others, including the farrowing house, the service area (especially for new gilts) and, to a lesser extent, the immediate post-weaning accommodation, all demand almost constant attention by a skilled stockman. This person must have ample time to observe and deal promptly with any problems and provide a stable and optimal environment to cater for the very different needs of the pigs in these three very critical areas of production.

FIVE STAGES

The approach to poor productivity in growing pigs will be covered under the five major stages of production used in contemporary intensive systems of bacon production. For each stage, an attempt will be made to provide a priority listing of factors that lead to poor productivity. However, it must be remembered that the ultimate controlling influence on production at every stage is management and this will have a direct bearing on productivity at each phase of the operation.

Optimal production in the growing pig implies:

(1)   Growth from birth to slaughter in as short a time as possible.
(2)   Development of a carcass that will command the best grading and acceptability to the consumer.
(3)   The best economic return possible undiluted by the cost of deaths, disease and medication.

The ability to obtain optimal production requires a multiplicity of factors. The most important of these are the ability of the manager to maximize the genetic potential of the particular type of pig in use, to control the in-house environment so as to maintain conditions that do not fluctuate, and to provide a diet that is best for the various ages of pig.

One cannot stress enough the role of management in obtaining optimal production. The physical condition of the floors, fittings and feeding systems, the type of food, regularity of feeding and dietary composition are all under the direct control of management. If these factors are not optimized, because of the lack of money or the poor performance of management, then production efficiency will be reduced accordingly, even to the point, in the worst case, of the unit being economically non-viable.

BIRTH TO WEANING

The aim, at the start of this period, should be to rear all pigs that are born alive. Having said this there will, on occasions, be piglets that at birth are very much underweight and will not survive beyond 1–2 days. If the frequency of this type of piglet is very high, then a detailed investigation will have to be made of the sow and its management during the previous lactation and during the whole of the dry period.

It is essential, with all litters, to ensure that there are adequate heating lamps, both at the rear of the sow and in the creep area, or under-floor heating to provide the right temperature for the newly born piglets. Cold, wet conditions will rapidly deplete energy reserves in the neonatal piglet and will severely compromise its survival. For similar reasons, draughts at or around floor level should be avoided.

The next most important factor is to ensure that there are enough functional teats for the number of piglets born. This step is often ignored until piglets are found dead from starvation 2–3 days after birth. Also, there is a need to ensure that the sow continues to produce adequate milk for the whole of the suckling period.

This scale of observation demands almost constant attention from the stockman in charge of the farrowing accommodation and failure to provide this attention will almost certainly result in either piglet deaths or low weaning weights.

Bacterial infections

Various bacterial infections may be seen during the suckling period, both in the sow and its offspring, which will affect the ultimate productivity of the litter. The most important conditions are those affecting the sow's udder.

Soon after farrowing, sows may develop a hot swollen udder, show signs of aggression and fail to eat. The piglets, as well as being deprived of adequate milk, may have diarrhoea and be constantly squealing. Attention is too often directed at the piglets with the sow being ignored until piglets have died and the sow has refused to eat for several days. The failure to recognize the real problem is very often due to lack of defined routines for the care of suckling sows or a failure to allocate adequate staff or time to this area of the operation. The type of mastitis just described is often seen with solid-floored farrowing pens having sawdust bedding that is perpetually wet with urine. Such a situation will yield ammonia that is toxic to the nipples and also high numbers of bacteria such as *Escherichia coli*, proteus and even klebsiella, all of which can damage the milk-laden udder.

Batch weaning

A procedure frequently leading to the initiation of poor productivity in sucking piglets is the common policy of batch weaning on a specific date. This technique would be highly desirable if all sows were to farrow on the same day. Unfortunately, this is not the case as there will frequently be at least 7 days difference between the first and last farrowing in a mixed group of 14–16 sows and gilts. Batch weaning of piglets from such a group will mean a spread of ages from 14 to 21 days with the younger age groups often being too immature to cope with the next stage of production which involves an abrupt conversion from a liquid milk diet to one of pellets and water. Recognition of this problem by management and the introduction of split-weaning with the younger, lighter-weight piglets being kept on good milking sows or in a controlled environment tent receiving a milk-based diet for a further 7 days before transfer, will usually solve the problem.

FIRST-STAGE FLAT DECK ACCOMMODATION

The initial productivity of piglets at this stage depends to a great extent on what has happened to them during the suckling period. If, for instance, batch weaning operates and all piglets are weaned irrespective of age, then a proportion of these piglets will arrive on the flat decks very immature in terms of the digestive tract and will have a difficult time competing with their more mature contemporaries. This situation produces the characteristic "fading piglet syndrome" in which the immature piglets cannot compete, cannot digest enough solid food and may not readily take to drinking water. These piglets, unless recognized quickly, very soon become anorexic and may die of a combination of dehydation and starvation.

The measures for preventing this syndrome have already been described in the foregoing section. Initially, there will be no problem from overcrowding but by the end of this first-stage growing period the individual pens can be heavily congested and if they are not emptied at the requisite time then not only does productivity suffer but also welfare is compromised and vices may appear.

Environmental control

The control of the environment in the first stage accommodation presents a major challenge to management, e.g.

(1) Temperature. A temperature very close to that found in the creep area has to be produced which later takes into account the increased production of body heat as the piglets mature. There is also the need later to reduce temperature on a regular basis to that which will be found in the second-stage growing area.
(2) Ventilation. This has to be increased proportionate to the growth rate of the piglets to regulate temperature and also to remove waste gases and excessive humidity.

Failure to regulate the environment properly could result in the piglets being too hot or too cold and to a dangerous build-up of noxious gases, especially carbon dioxide or carbon monoxide, if inefficient gas heaters are used. A situation might also be produced that would permit the survival of pathogenic agents in moist air and allow the widespread distribution of dust particles that would act as an irritant to the upper respiratory tract.

It is particularly important at this point of growth to provide piglets with an environment in which they are content. If such an environment is not provided then the uncomfortable conditions will probably lead to the initiation of vices such as tail- and ear-biting. Also, certain environment-associated infections such as exudative epidermitis (greasy pig disease) will be more prevalent in an unpleasant humid environment than one which is pleasant and fresh. This disease can also be initiated by fighting after mixing, by sharp projections on floors and metal fittings and also from wounds inflicted by biting flies. The effect on productivity can be disastrous in that in severe outbreaks up to 75% of all piglets in a house can be affected. Once established, the disease is difficult to halt and many piglets will die of dehydration and electrolyte loss despite heroic attempts at treatment.

Other causes of poor production during the first-stage growth period are respiratory infections such as atrophic rhinitis (Fig. 2.1), haemophilus and mycoplasma pneumonias. The maintenance of a suitable microclimate within the flat deck accommodation is essential to keep down the air-borne spread of pathogens. As mentioned already, the stock density should not result in overcrowding as this is one of the main contributory factors to the infection of piglets with agents causing respiratory disease.

SECOND-STAGE FLATS

Some of the problems occurring in the first-stage flat decks will be readily transferred to the second-stage accommodation. These include piglets with bitten tails and/or chronic respiratory infection. Several of these will not thrive in the new conditions and will die or have to be destroyed thus seriously affecting productivity at this stage of growth. Of special concern are the possible effects of tail biting (Fig. 2.2) as very often after the initial injury the primary lesion may heal. If infection had occurred then it would probably penetrate into the deeper tissues often passing up the spinal column to produce one or more abscesses leading to pressure on the spinal cord with resultant hind quarter lameness and possibly paralysis (Fig. 2.3). Since the paralysis cannot be relieved, destruction of the pig results in a loss of production from the amount of feed it has consumed and also loss of the marketable value of the carcass.

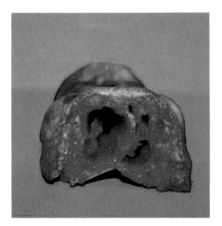

Fig. 2.1
Section of pig's snout showing evidence of atrophic rhinitis.

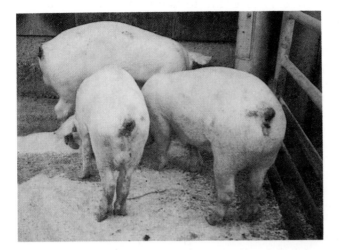

Fig. 2.2
Pigs showing
evidence of tail
biting.

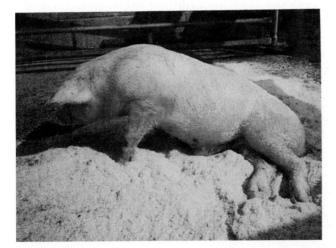

Fig. 2.3
Pig with hind quarter
paralysis.

Microclimate

As with other areas of accommodation, the microclimate must be maintained at a stable level suitable for the particular age group of pig. Failure to regulate the environment properly can lead to serious losses in production. If the temperature is too high losses will occur from unnecessary use of energy and although a high temperature may be being used in an attempt to reduce feed uptake, the cost of this exercise probably would not justify its use. Conversely, if the temperature is too cold in an attempt to save on energy costs the pigs will be uncomfortable, many of them will pass very loose faeces and the whole area and its pigs will soon be very dirty. The uptake of food in an *ad libitum* situation will be higher than necessary under cold conditions in an attempt to increase body heat production and with rationed food intake cold pigs will very soon lose weight as food will be directed to heat production rather than protein deposition. Over the long term either the extra cost of electrical energy or the loss in daily live weight gain will lead to a serious reduction in production (= profitability) of the unit.

Floors

A further feature in the environment that will lead to a falling off in production relates to the type and condition of the floors present in the pens. In one type of system, pen floors may consist of slats made of concrete or metal with or without a non-slatted area in front of the feeding troughs. It is essential that the gap between the slats is appropriate for the size of pig being housed. If too large, then feet, hocks and elbows can enter the gap and the skin and underlying tissues become damaged producing initially painful hygromatous swellings which may then be infected and lead to abscesses or even septic arthritis (Fig. 2.4). Also, the pigs will be uncomfortable and this often leads to continuing tail and ear biting. Damage to the tissues overlying the joints at this stage will cause loss of productivity later on when gilts will be rejected at selection because of leg damge and/or subcutaneous abscesses.

Prolapse of the rectum

Prolapse of the rectum (Fig. 2.5) is a problem often seen in second-stage flat decks especially with overcrowded conditions where pigs tend to lie on top of each other or when there is an outbreak of enteritis. If seen early it can be surgically treated but often the prolapsed section gets chewed by other

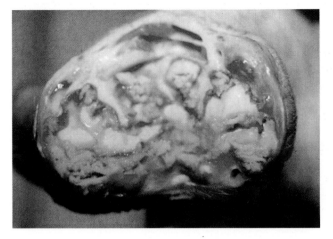

Fig. 2.4
Leg joint showing
septic arthritis.

pigs and on healing there will be scarring and stricture of the rectum (Fig. 2.6). Since the pig will be unable to pass normal faeces a characteristic rectal stricture syndrome is produced with the affected pig losing a lot of weight, having a very swollen abdomen and failing to develop (Fig. 2.7). Such pigs are a total loss to the system with a consequent loss of profitability.

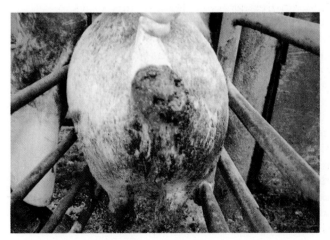

Fig. 2.5
Hind quarter of a
bacon type pig
showing rectal
prolapse.

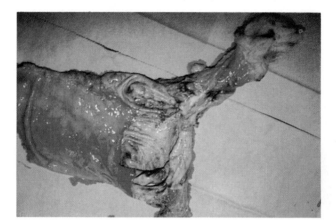

Fig. 2.6
Ballooning of the
hind gut with scarring
and stricture of the
rectum.

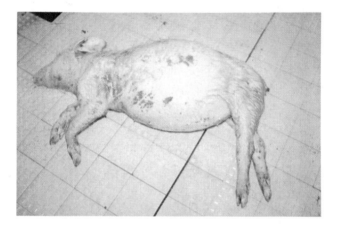

Fig. 2.7
Rectal stricture
syndrome with the
affected pig showing
loss of condition and
a very swollen
abdomen.

STRAW YARD OR PRE-FINISH ACCOMMODATION

As with previous stages there will be a carry over of problems such as tail biting, leg lesions and, to a lesser extent, ear and flank biting. Fortunately, the conditions in most pre-finish accommodation do permit more space per pig than was allowed indoors in the second-stage flat deck accommodation. This has several advantages in that pigs can get away from a "bully" especially if the pen is longer than it is wide; if the pens are outdoors with a kennel area then deficiencies in the environment become less of a problem. Many of the difficulties in this pre-finish accommodation result from lack of observation by the stockman who, because of automatic feeding and watering, may only glance at those pigs that he can see at best once per day.

If automatic pipeline feeding is used great care must be taken to ensure that blockages do not occur, with pigs being deprived of food for several days. The same reasoning applies especially during winter when freezing of the water supply will inevitably lead to deaths and loss of production because of salt poisoning.

Production will also suffer if inefficient observers fail to detect early signs of ill health especially meningitis, pneumonia and enteritis. Most of these conditions, if seen early, will respond favourably to medication but if treatment is delayed the disease may have progressed too far for recovery to occur.

Floors

The condition of the floors can seriously affect production. Failure to replace or repair damaged concrete or wire slats can result in pigs falling through the damaged area and drowning in the slurry pit. Less apparent damage, especially of weld mesh or wire floors, often results in multiple injuries to the feet and legs. This can lead to septic arthritis or even vegetative endocarditis from the entry of bacteria through permanently damaged skin causing a bacteraemia with localization of bacteria on the heart valves.

Waste foods

Under conditions of poor economic gain, sub-standard batches of feed or waste human foods may be purchased at low cost in an attempt to improve unit profitability. Such feed may be low in nutrients, contain high levels of mycotoxins or be of a nature totally unsuitable for pig feeding. It is essential with fast growing pigs to provide a standard diet at regular intervals. Only in this way is it possible to obtain efficient weight gain and feed conversion consistently.

Disease

Disease problems at this stage of growth are minimal unless, of course, replacements are purchased from a variety of sources including livestock markets. Under these conditions each new batch of pigs brought on to the unit may well be carrying a variety of disease-causing agents whose spread around the unit will cause serious losses in production and may even result in the epidemic spread of a pathogen causing many pigs to become ill and die. As with all other stages of production, pigs will only grow as well as the environment and management permit.

FINAL FINISHER PHASE

The performance and hence productivity of pigs at this stage are essentially indicators of the quality of management. Accepting that rapidly growing hybrids are used in the first instance their ultimate performance will depend upon the type and quality of feed, the environment in which they are kept, and the application of good managemental routines.

Disease also plays a part at this stage of the production cycle but an understanding manager can adjust the environment to ensure that the best conditions are produced to prevent the flare up of diseases which, previously, have been kept under rigid control. All chronically sick animals should have been recognized and disposed of during the early phases of growth.

Overcrowding

There are, however, many deficiencies that can occur in this final stage of production. Overcrowding is generally one of the most common faults and is probably a result of upper management simply playing the numbers game. With this philosophy the environmental, biological and welfare needs of the pig are ignored and the measures implemented to increase or maintain profitability in fact have the opposite effect. The net result of increasing the number of pigs per pen is to increase the time taken to reach slaughter weight and the grade of carcass produced is also reduced. The number of pigs per pen in the final stage of growth must be carefully adjusted to ensure optimal growth of each pig. Generally speaking, it is better to have one fewer pig in the pen than one more. The days to market will improve and the group as a whole will perform better. With overcrowding each pen will contain one or more pigs lighter in weight which have to be sold out of contract or be retained on the unit for a further period of time with all the attendant problems of managing a number of individual animals.

As the pigs reach finishing weight it is essential to ensure appropriate control of ventilation. Frequently the fans or louvres are set at the start of the period and remain at this setting instead of being adjusted to cope with the fluctuations of weather and the changes that occur from night to day time.

Diet

The other factors that generally cause persistent problems are related to the nature and frequency of the diet. Economics of pig rearing demand that advantage be taken of seasonal availability of milk products but the sudden introduction of skim or whey into the diet produces a series of health problems which can result in the death of many pigs.

Sudden bloat with death is commonly associated with whey feeding and it is now recognized that any upset of the intestinal bacteria, such as that caused by the abrupt introduction of skim milk, can result in the overgrowth of intestinal bacteria such as campylobacters which produce dysentery-like signs. The same also applies when skim is suddenly withdrawn and replaced by cereals.

Many other factors associated with feeding, such as wet or dry meal, *ad libitum* or restricted feeding, and two or three feeds per day, should be investigated when trying to optimize growth and carcass quality. The introduction of computerized pipeline feeding has produced its own problems such as unrecognized pipeline blockages, reluctance of management to ensure that the pigs are actually getting the requisite quantity of feed, and, in particular, the failure to reduce the amount of feed delivered to a pen when a pig dies or is removed for other reasons.

Losses

Finally, health problems that started at earlier stages in the growing cycle often result in deaths in the finishing house. This applies particularly to conditions like vegetative endocarditis stemming from chronic leg lesions being infected with strepto-coccal organisms and also persistent pleurisy associated with previous haemophilus infections. Losses at this final stage of production are very serious in that there is no casualty payment and the pig has cost a considerable sum of money to rear it almost to market weight.

Extensive units

Many of the problems with production in intensive systems apply equally to extensively managed units. There are, how-ever, specific situations which have a direct application to extensive units. There is a particular need to recognize the effect of extremes of weather on outdoor pig health and productivity. Parasites, both external and internal, are a persistent problem for outdoor pigs.

There is also a need to provide wallows in hot weather and to appreciate the effect of sharp flintstones in the soil causing damage to the udder and feet. Of particular importance is the need to ensure that outdoor pigs get their full ration of food, that boars are not allowed too many services and especially that they do not direct all their serving energy to one favourite sow or gilt.

Diseases such as cystitis or pyelonephritis require rapid recognition and treatment; the same also applies to breeding failures, which should be recognized and investigated as soon as possible. As with indoor intensive systems, frequent observation by competent stockmen is essential to avoid any delay in the detection and treatment of health and welfare problems.

CONCLUSION

It is patently obvious that the production problems described above result directly or indirectly from some action of management. These include failure to impose security precautions, improper control of temperature and ventilation systems, bad maintenance of fixtures such as slatted floors and concrete areas, and problems associated with feeding and feeding systems. Finally, many production problems can also be caused by upper or executive management imposing routines or procedures based solely on budget or financial considerations.

CHAPTER 3

Penile Injuries in the Boar

CHRISTIANNE GLOSSOP

INTRODUCTION

Penile injuries in the boar are only rarely drawn to the attention of the veterinary surgeon and for this reason are not usually considered of any great significance. Most injuries under the broad heading of "bleeding boar" are treated by conservative means only and although such cases often recover, the occasional failures can represent a significant loss to the pig producer. The effect of such injuries on fertility, combined with the escalating cost of replacing top performance tested boars, has led to an increased demand on the part of the breeder for detailed examination and treatment of valuable sires. In addition, experienced handling of boars and supervision during service are essential to minimize the risk of injury.

In an attempt to outline the general principles of approaching penile injury and treatment of the various conditions, it is necessary to remind ourselves of the functional anatomy of the boar penis.

ANATOMY

The boar penis is fibroelastic in structure, consisting of two main cavernous bodies surrounded by a collagenous tunica albuginea (Fig. 3.1). The tunica albuginea in the boar is significantly thinner than it is in the bull. The corpus cavernosum penis surrounds the urethra dorsally and laterally. It is markedly vascular with a profusion of cavernous spaces arranged around a framework of fine trabeculae. The large cavernous spaces are primarily longitudinal in direction.

The urethra lies in a ventral position, completely surrounded by a second cavernous body, the corpus spongiosum penis. These cavernous spaces are large, especially dorsal to the urethra, where one main vascular cavity is traversed by long narrow trabeculae. Both the corpus cavernosum and the corpus spongiosum penis extend along the length of the organ, from the root to the free end. There appear to be no vascular connections between the two cavernous bodies. There is no distinct glans penis in the boar. The corpus spongiosum

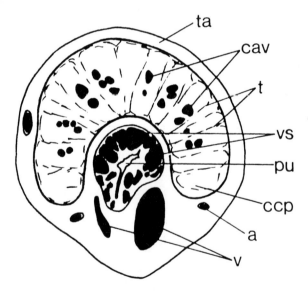

Fig. 3.1 Diagram of transverse section of the free part of the boar penis. The corpus cavernosum penis (ccp) contains large longitudinal cavernous spaces (cav). The corpus spongiosum penis surrounds the penile urethra (pu): it shows large vascular spaces (vs); veins (v) lie deep to and arteries (a) lie superficial to the tunica albuginea (ta) which surrounds both cavernous bodies.

glandis is described only as a venous plexus in the skin covering the tip of the penis. There is evidence of a direct vascular connection between the corpus spongiosum penis and the corpus spongiosum glandis via fine cavernous spaces at the urethral orifice.

The root of the penis is surrounded by the striated ischiocavernosus and bulbospongiosus muscles. The body of the penis runs along the ventral abdomen, supported by penile fascia and skin; it forms a sigmoid flexure cranial to the scrotum. The free end is that part of the penis occupying the caudal section of the preputial cavity when the penis is fully retracted (Fig. 3.2). The free end is covered by the penile integument and is the part most commonly involved in injuries. It describes a spiral shape at rest with the characteristic three-and-a-quarter to three-and-three-quarter twists which become more marked at erection. The cranial section of the preputial cavity communicates with a dorsal diverticulum which contains a putrid liquid.

INDICATIONS FOR EXAMINATION OF THE PENIS

REDUCTION IN FERTILITY (WITH OR WITHOUT LOSS OF LIBIDO)

Records must be examined in order to identify a subfertile boar, particularly on a commercial unit where two different sires are often used on the same sow during one oestrous

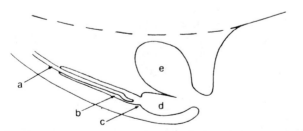

Fig. 3.2 Lateral view of the penis (a) lying in the caudal section of the preputial cavity (b). The preputial diverticulum (e) opens into the cranial section of the preputial cavity (d) dorsally. A ridge (c) divides the preputial cavity into the two sections.

period. Age of boar, previous service behaviour, farrowing
rate and litter size should be considered.

HISTORY OF TRAUMA

Accidents resulting in penile injury most commonly occur
during mating or masturbation. Observation of haematuria,
or haemospermia during mating, are indicative of injury.

In all cases, examination of the penis should be carried out
in conjunction with a complete examination of the external
genitalia. It is also helpful to observe the boar's sexual
behaviour in the usual service pen.

Under normal circumstances, a boar introduced to an
oestrous sow should first of all exhibit pre-copulatory behaviour – salivation, nuzzling and biting the female, followed by
attempts to mount. Hesistance at this stage may indicate pain
associated with erection or copulation. Having mounted the
sow, erection and protrusion of the free end of the penis will
precede thrusting movements as the boar searches for the
vulva. This presents an ideal opportunity for inspection of the
penis, as most of the free end will protrude from the preputial
orifice. Failure of erection at this stage may indicate impotence
or other penile abnormalities.

The surface of the penis should be examined for abrasions,
lacerations and ulcerations. Haemorrhage from one or both
cavernous bodies will be exacerbated by erection and the
site of injury will be more easily identified. Any fertility
examination on a boar should include the collection of an
ejaculate and this also facilitates a closer inspection of the
penis. Once it has mounted, the boar should be approached
from the rear and the gloved hand placed immediately cranial
to the urethral orifice, with the back of the hand against the
ventral abdomen. Gentle pressure should be applied to the
distal few centimetres until the penis locks into the hand
which mimics the spiral folds of the sow's cervix. Ejaculation
can take 5–10 min and a detailed examination of the free end
of the penis and the site of the preputial reflection is possible
at this time.

If an injury is identified which appears to require anything
more than the simplest of treatments, passive exposure of the
penis is necessary. A wide range of anaesthetics is available

for this purpose; experience from practice indicates that a reliable method is a combination of azaperone and metomidate hydrochloride (Stresnil and Hypnodil; Janssen) which produces a state of general anaesthesia accompanied by good muscle relaxation. The boar should be kept as calm and quiet as possible during the induction and recovery periods.

Partial erection may accompany barbiturate induced anaesthesia and this will simplify penile exposure. The penis is eased out of the prepuce by pushing the shaft cranially and everting the preputial mucosa. Once the tip becomes visible it should be held firmly by a gloved hand (this procedure can be time-consuming); this facilitates detailed examination of penile integument, the urethral orifice and the preputial reflection.

INJURIES TO THE PENIS

SUPERFICIAL WOUNDS

The tip of the penis is the most common site for abrasions and contusions (Fig. 3.3). These may occur as a result of clumsy or inexperienced mating, or masturbation. Ulcerations are most often found at the preputial reflection (Fig. 3.4) and may be the site of intermittent haemorrhage. Minor injuries are generally incidental findings, causing slight pain and discomfort during mating but rarely influencing fertility. Two to three weeks rest may be advised, with broad spectrum antibiotic therapy if the injuries are extensive.

DEEP WOUNDS

Puncture wounds and lacerations also occur at mating or during masturbation, or during attempts to escape from the pen. It is suggested that inexperienced boars may be injured when the erect penis comes into contact with the sow's bristles. Deep wounds may penetrate one of the cavernous bodies and result in extensive haemorrhage which is more marked during erection and ejaculation (Figs 3.5 and 3.6). When erection is not impaired, fertility may be reduced in

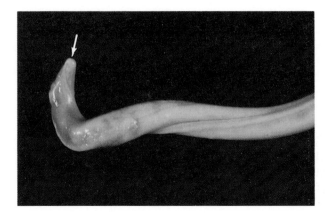

Fig. 3.3
Free end of the boar penis: note the spiral arrangement even at rest. The urethral orifice is shown (arrow).

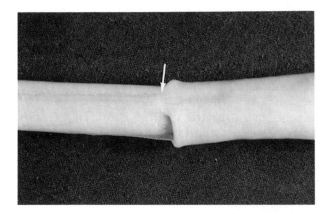

Fig. 3.4
The preputial reflection (arrow) is a common site of ulceration (the penis is on the left).

some instances as a result of haemospermia.

If the site of the injury is visible, surgical repair may be undertaken under general anaesthesia. The penis should be exposed as described and washed with saline or a mild solution of cetrimide (Cetavlon; ICI). Haemorrhage may be controlled by a tourniquet. Rough jagged edges should be trimmed with pointed scissors. A continuous eversion suture pattern should be employed using self-threaded Dexon (Davis & Geck) on an atraumatic needle. If the wound is small, a purse-string suture may be sufficient. Cautery of small lesions is rarely successful. Following repair the penis should be

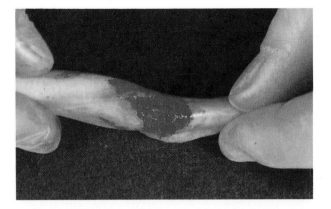

Fig. 3.5
Abrasions and deep laceration penetrating the corpus cavernosum penis approximately 8 cm distal to the preputial reflection.

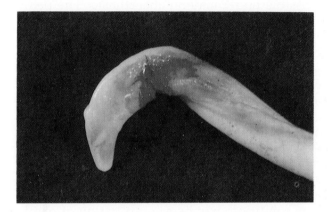

Fig. 3.6
Severe damage to the free end of the penis, involving both cavernous bodies and the urethra.

lubricated with an oil-based antibiotic and eased back into the prepuce. Postoperative management is imperative to the success of treatment (see later).

If damage to the cavernous bodies is extensive it may not be possible to repair the wound successfully. Alternatively, fine blood vessels may develop at the site of the repair resulting in impotence caused by distal venous drainage; this condition therefore carries a guarded prognosis. Fistulation of the urethra as a result of external trauma or urolithiasis can result in haematuria or haemospermia. There is no treatment possible for such damage to the cavernous bodies as the site is inaccessible to surgical repair. On occasion the spiral tip of the penis may be bitten off when an inexperienced boar mounts the head end of the sow. Under these circumstances a boar is usually rendered infertile since a lock cannot be achieved during copulation. Such an animal is not necessarily impotent: a small number of cases are recorded in which the damaged end of the penis heals of its own accord.

PROLAPSED PENIS

As seen in other species, penile prolapse in the boar occasionally follows treatment with neuroleptics. The penis may become congested, contused and abraded and should be protected from further injury by wrapping in a damp towel until treatment is commenced. Treatment should be carried out as soon as possible under general anaesthesia. The penis should be washed and wounds repaired. Lubricating the surface with an oily antibiotic suspension will aid reduction of the prolapse. The penis is eased into the caudal section of the preputial cavity.

A purse-string suture at the preputial orifice will avoid the risk of repeated prolapse. Balanoposthitis is a possible complication of penile prolapse so it is wise to employ postoperative topical and systemic antibiotic therapy.

PROLAPSED PREPUCE

This relatively rare condition may be a complication of penile prolapse. In a mild case, the exposed tissues should be cleaned with a mild solution of warm cetrimide, the oedema reduced by pressure and the prolapsed mucosa eased back into the sheath. Prognosis in such simple cases is generally good. In cases of longer standing, the tissues are usually oedematous and traumatized and when the preputial mucosa is badly damaged resection is usually necessary. This procedure is possible provided that the entrance to the preputial diverticulum is intact.

Under general anaesthesia the prolapse is eased cranially and the skin of the preputial orifice caudally in order to expose intact mucosa. The prolapse is fixed using a padded artery clamp to keep the stump exteriorized following resection. Two catgut threads are run crosswise through the prolapsed tube of the mucosa before the affected tissue is removed. The threads are then cut so as to provide four separate stay sutures which are tied. At least eight more sutures are then placed along the edges of the stump. The clamp is removed and the line of sutures eased back into the prepuce.

MANAGEMENT

Careful management of boars is essential to recovery following penile injury. The points listed below form a general guideline for postoperative treatment:

(1)   Keep the boar isolated and well bedded-down.
(2)   Reflex excitability may be reduced by administration of azaperone (Stresnil; Janssen) for the first few days following surgery. This should only be employed if absolutely necessary as penile prolapse may follow. In feed, preparations to reduce excitability in pigs are on trial at the present time (e.g. amperozide which is a new psychotropic compound (Andersson *et al.*, 1986): these may provide a useful alternative to an injectable sedative.
(3)   Where haemorrhage is severe, promote coagulation of blood by administration of calcium solution and vitamin K.
(4)   Allow the boar 4 weeks rest before sexual activity.
(5)   Supervise natural service and hand-mate if necessary, particularly for the first few services after treatment. Adhesions forming around the site of the injury may result in discomfort during copulation.

It should be recognized that boars require careful training and good management, particularly at service, and that these should reduce the incidence of penile injuries which, although relatively uncommon, may have a serious effect on the fertility of individual boars.

REFERENCES

Andersson, K., Hiödversson, R. & Göransson, R. (1986). *Proceedings of the 9th International Pig Veterinary Society Conference, Barcelona.*

CHAPTER 4

Pregnancy Diagnosis in Pigs

MICHAEL MEREDITH

INTRODUCTION

Pig producers often turn to veterinarians for advice on pregnancy diagnosis. Their most common request is to identify non-pregnant pigs as soon as possible after service, so that they can be quickly re-mated or culled and replaced. This is quite understandable considering that the cost of keeping an empty sow (including loss of production) is £11–£16 per week.

Routine pregnancy testing is not always cost effective, however. All pregnancy tests produce occasional errors – more than occasional with some of the cheaper tests! False negative results on pregnant sows are particularly costly and few people have sufficient confidence in their pregnancy test to cull a sow on the basis of a single negative result. What usually happens is that these sows are retained for further testing and checking for return to oestrus. This both reduces the economic value of prompt action on an initial negative result and increases the real cost of detecting non-pregnant sows.

Even in situations where routine pregnancy testing is not cost-effective, producers may still wish to undertake it because of the greater managemental control or peace of mind that it offers.

In addition to advising on pregnancy tests, some veterinarians find that personal skill in pregnancy testing can be of value for regular fertility-monitoring work and in the investigation of reproductive problems.

There are many potential applications of pregnancy testing and no test is universally superior (Table 4.1). In each situation the economic, convenience and accuracy factors have to be taken into account in deciding if pregnancy testing will be worthwhile and which test to use. Judicious usage requires an understanding of the features and limitations of the range of tests available.

PREGNANCY TESTS

Many techniques have been devised for determining the pregnancy status of pigs, but few have survived close examination of their accuracy, cost and practical feasibility. The techniques listed in Table 4.2 and described below are those that are currently worthy of consideration.

NON-RETURN TO OESTRUS

This is undoubtedly the most widely used criterion of pregnancy status. Detecting returns in non-pregnant pigs can be considered to be a continuous process from service to farrowing, but in practice the most significant efforts are often concentrated into a limited period when returns are most likely to occur, e.g. 18–25 days after service. Accuracy varies widely depending largely on the extent to which a boar is used and on the type of housing (Meredith, 1980). Cost-saving housing for dry sows may impair detection of returns to the extent that considerable time and money has to be spent on special pregnancy tests.

Detection of returns may be used as a preliminary screening test whereby only those pigs that have not returned by a particular time are subjected to a special pregnancy test. It may also be used to confirm the negative findings of a previous special test, e.g. negative sows are retained in the service area until a return is detected.

Table 4.1 Potential applications of pregnancy testing

Routine use

Testing all sows at a short interval (e.g. 3–4 weeks) after service to detect empty sows for re-mating/treatment/culling

Confirmation of pregnancy before moving from service area to pregnancy accommodation

Checking any sows suspected of being "not-in-pig" at a later stage (2–3 months) after service

Regular monitoring of pregnancy rate for early detection of infertility. It may be sufficient to test only a proportion of mated sows

Forecasting future production (planning output, accommodation, etc.). It may be sufficient to test only a proportion of mated sows

Occasional use

Identifying pregnant pigs when service records or ear tags are lost

Identification of pregnant pigs after unsupervised contact with boar

Confirmation of pregnancy in animals to be sold as "in-pig"

Detection of retained fetuses in cases of dystocia

To assist decisions regarding treatment or culling of casualty sows

In the investigation of infertility problems, determining:

Impact of problem on productivity and profitability

Epidemiology of problem, e.g. stage of gestation affected

Which pigs to subject to diagnostic investigations

Exclusion of pregnancy in cases of anoestrus

EXTERNAL PHYSICAL SIGNS

As pregnancy advances, enlargement of the ventral abdomen and udder become noticeable. In parous sows the skin over the mammae is very wrinkled but these wrinkles disappear as pregnancy progresses. In gilts, enlargement of the teats is a prominent feature (Fig. 4.1) In the last month of pregnancy, fetal movements can be seen when sows are lying quietly. Finally, in the last 2 weeks of pregnancy, there is a progressive flabby enlargement of the vulva.

Checking for these late confirmatory signs of pregnancy should be a routine part of management to detect sows which were either false positives in an earlier pregnancy test or were true positives which have subsequently suffered pregnancy failure. Possible negatives revealed at this inspection can be re-tested.

Table 4.2 Comparison of pregnancy tests

Test	Days after service			Costs[a]	% Accuracy on pigs that[b]		Main sources of errors		Special merits or problems
	Earliest	Latest	Optimum		Farrow	Do not farrow	False +[c]	False −	
A-mode ultrasound	23	85	30–70	£200–£1025 for instrument	63–99	40–96	Bladder Uterine pus/semen Ovarian cysts	Inadequate scanning Scatter/absorption by gut contents	Quick, easy test
Blood progesterone	17	Term	17–20	£1 per sow	97–100 (ELISA)	60–78	Delayed returns Pseudo-pregnancy	Assay errors	
Doppler ultrasound Uterine artery Pulse	21	Term	30–40	£250–£350 for instrument	83–100	60–99	Endometritis Pro-oestrus/ oestrus Other maternal arteries	Inadequate scanning	Prolonged use distressing to ears
Fetal pulse	28	Term	42–term		62–100[d]	89–100[d]	Rapid maternal pulse	Inadequate scanning	Confirmation of fetal viability. Prediction of farrowing date

External physical signs	42	Term	>55(gilts) >84(sows)	Negligible	82–100	no data	Recently fed Pseudo-pregnancy[c] Obesity	Small litters Individual varn.	Cheap confirmation of late pregnancy
Non-return to oestrus[f]	Daily 18–24	–	Daily 18–30	Suitable housing	98–100	25–94	Inactive ovaries Delayed returns Pseudo-pregnancy[e] Poor detection of oestrus	Too ill or too restricted to resist mounting	Oestrus detection necessary anyway if empty sows to be re-mated
Oestrone sulphate	18	77–term	25–29	£1 per sow (ELISA)	94–100	65–100		Small litters	Useful to diagnose death of embryos
Real-time ultrasound	19	Term	24–term	£5000–£10 000 for instrument	100	61–100	Uterine pus/semen Ovarian cysts	Inadequate scanning	Can detect mummified fetuses. Fetal age/health information. Needs 240 V lead

continued

Table 4.2 Continued

Test	Days after service			Costs[a]	% Accuracy on pigs that[b]		Main sources of errors		Special merits or problems
	Earliest	Latest	Optimum		Farrow	Do not farrow	False +[c]	False −	
Rectal palpation									
Cervix	18	Term	18–21		100	44–57			Gilts too small
Uterine artery	21	Term	28–term		99–100	86–94	Endometritis Fremitus from external iliac artery	Artery to bladder palpated in error	Gynaecological examination of negative sows possible
All features	18	Term	30–term		95–100	94–100			

[a]Wholesale prices excluding VAT. Labour cost to be added.
[b]Accuracy relates to a single test undertaken by competent personnel at optimum time after service. Figures quoted are the range of sensitivities (accuracy on sows that later farrow or abort) and specificities (accuracy on sows not subsequently farrowing) in recent trials. Doubtful results counted as errors.
[c]Pregnancy failure after testing produces false positives.
[d]Refers to fetal pulse alone. If uterine artery included, accuracy is higher on pregnant and lower on non-pregnant pigs.
[e]Can be caused by mycotoxin or follow mummification of entire litter.
[f]Daily detection of oestrus with a boar.

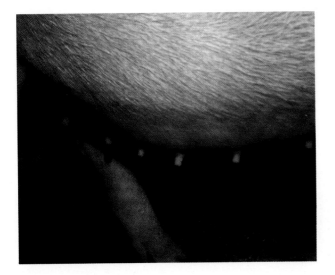

Fig. 4.1
Enlargement of teats, mammary tissue and lower abdomen in a pregnant gilt, 3 months after service.

DOPPLER ULTRASOUND

The abdomen is scanned with an ultrasound beam emitted from an external hand-held transducer (rectal probes are also available, but less convenient). The same transducer is receptive to reflections of this beam. If the reflections are from moving structures they will have suffered a frequency change and are converted to audible sounds via headphones or a loudspeaker (Fig. 4.2). With all ultrasound techniques it is important to have the sows reasonably still to facilitate scanning, and this is particularly the case with the Doppler technique. It usually takes only 1–2 min per sow to detect positive sounds but negative conclusions may require a rather longer search (from both flanks) to be reliable.

The type of sound which can be detected earliest in pregnancy originates from increased blood flow in the uterine arteries. Pulsatile sounds from these vessels are rarely detected in non-pregnant pigs. In pregnant pigs the sounds may occasionally appear as early as 3 weeks after service, but negative findings are unreliable until about 4 weeks. Whenever the scanning results on one side of a pig are negative it is advisable to check from the other side too (the two arteries may differ in blood flow and also it is easy to miss such a small structure when scanning with a narrow beam).

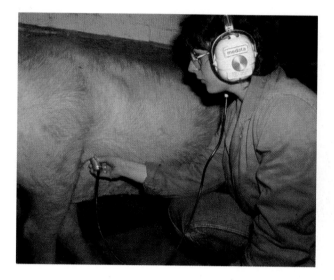

Fig. 4.2
Auscultation of
uterine artery sounds
with a Doppler
ultrasound
instrument.

From about the sixth week of pregnancy it is possible to detect pulsations of the fetal heart and umbilical vessels. These pulsatile sounds are twice or three times the rate of the resting maternal pulse and provide much more specific evidence of pregnancy. Fetal movements can be detected in the last month of pregnancy but are unreliable for diagnostic purposes.

A-MODE (PULSE-ECHO/AMPLITUDE-DEPTH) ULTRASOUND

This type of ultrasound scanning differs from the Doppler technique in that it is the amplitude (as opposed to frequency) of reflected sound which is detected. Reflections are particularly marked wherever the scanning beam encounters a solid/liquid interface. Thus marked reflections arise from the boundaries of fetal fluid in the pregnant uterus but they can also arise from other fluid-containing structures, particularly the bladder.

Potentially significant reflections can be displayed in a variety of ways: as an audible tone, light-emitting diode(s) or as an oscilloscope trace. Oscilloscope instruments (Fig. 4.3) are the most expensive and fragile, but allow a more sophisticated interpretation of reflections. Some instruments can also be

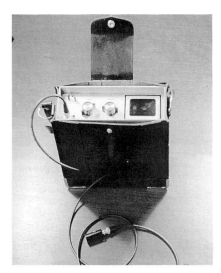

Fig. 4.3
An A-mode ultrasound instrument with oscilloscope display.

used for measuring thickness of backfat.

As with all ultrasound scanning, training and practice are important if high accuracy is to be achieved. A notable limitation of the A-mode test is that it is only reliable during the period when fetal fluid volume is significant, i.e. 25–70 days after service. It does have the advantage of requiring less restraint than other ultrasound techniques (Fig. 4.4). Scanning will usually take less than 1 min.

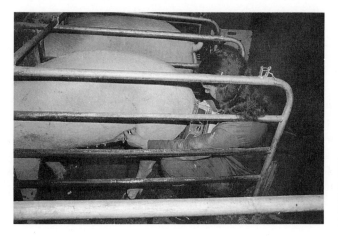

Fig. 4.4
Pregnancy testing with an A-mode (oscilloscope) ultrasound instrument.

REAL-TIME (B-MODE) ULTRASOUND

These instruments produce a moving cross-sectional image of tissue interfaces in the abdominal area that is scanned. Two main types are available: the linear array scanner (rectangular image) and the sector scanner (sectoral image). The latter has the advantage of requiring a smaller area of skin contact with the transducer. In early pregnancy the embryonic vesicles show up as irregular dark areas on the image. The embryos can be seen as white structures within these dark areas from about day 25 of pregnancy.

BLOOD PROGESTERONE

This test used to be expensive and require sophisticated laboratory facilities, but simple enzyme immunoassay kits are now available (Fig. 4.5). A single drop of blood from an ear vein is all that is required. The blood sample is obtained 17–20 days after service in order to distinguish between the high progesterone of maintained luteal function and the decline in progesterone which usually occurs in non-pregnant sows at this time. The test takes about 45 min to perform, once the samples have been collected. The labour involved will be considerable if only a few sows are tested at one time and this will lead to a high cost per pig tested.

The test can be used at later stages of pregnancy but only negative results will be reliable – positives can be obtained from sows in the luteal phase of a cycle. It is also useful for determining whether or not luteal tissue is present in cases of anoestrus.

OESTRONE SULPHATE

Pig embryos synthesize oestrogens, which are transformed into oestrone sulphate by the uterus and then enter the maternal circulation. A peak concentration in blood occurs between days 23 and 30 after service. Thereafter the concentration declines before rising again at around day 70. Radioimmunoassay of serum oestrone sulphate is a long and expensive procedure but an enzyme immunoassay kit is now

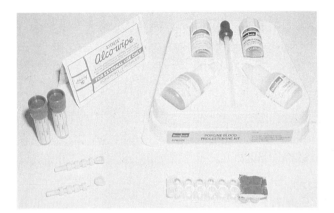

Fig. 4.5
An enzyme
immunoassay kit for
measuring blood
progesterone
concentration.

available and works on a single drop of whole blood.

This test is very specific and can be used to diagnose death of embryos in cases where positive sows subsequently become negative.

RECTAL PALPATION

Palpation of the genital tract *per rectum* is an invaluable technique for porcine fertility work, but surprisingly few veterinarians are familiar with it (Fig. 4.6). It does require some practice and care is necessary in handling the rectum and colon. The uterus is difficult to reach because it hangs low in the abdomen, but good diagnostic information can be obtained from the uterine arteries, cervix or ovaries.

The earliest signs of pregnancy can be detected at 3 weeks after service: persistence of corpora lutea and a cervix of soft consistency. In pigs that return to heat the cervix undergoes a remarkable thickening and hardening, beginning a couple of days before oestrus and continuing for a day or two afterwards. From about 1 month after service, uterine enlargement can be detected indirectly by the increasing tension on the cervix and broad ligaments; the ovaries are pulled progressively lower in the abdomen until they are out of reach.

The uterine arteries undergo enlargement and develop fremitus during pregnancy. They can be easily palpated within

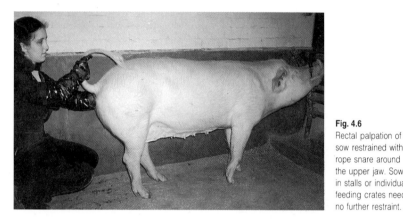

Fig. 4.6
Rectal palpation of a
sow restrained with a
rope snare around
the upper jaw. Sows
in stalls or individual
feeding crates need
no further restraint.

the pelvis and can be used as a rapid screening test for
pregnancy – negative pigs receiving a more extensive palpation
to confirm non-pregnancy and ascertain the functional state
of the ovaries. Fremitus can be induced (by slow occlusion)
in the uterine arteries of pregnant pigs from 4 weeks after
service.

Palpation of the genital tract is often impossible in gilts,
because of their small pelvis. The vaginal arteries are often
accessible in these cases, but enlargement and fremitus of
these vessels is not usually apparent until the last month of
pregnancy. Clinicians with large hands may have difficulty in
reaching the ovaries of primiparous sows.

ECONOMICS OF PREGNANCY TESTING

Table 4.3 gives some worked examples showing the economics
of pregnancy testing.

WHAT ACCURACY CAN WE EXPECT?

No pregnancy test can ever be 100% accurate over a substantial
number of pigs – if for no other reason than human errors
occasionally creeping in. Different trials of the same pregnancy

Table 4.3 Some worked examples showing economics of pregnancy testing

Description	Herd A Good performance	Herd B Poor detection of returns	Herd C Poor fertility	Calculation
Farrowing rate	85%	85%	75%	a
Efficiency of detecting returns	95%	80%	95%	b
Total services considered	1000	1000	1000	c
Number non-farrowing sows	150	150	250	$c(100-a)/100 = d$
Number non-farrowing sows cyclic by 4 weeks	120	120	200	$80\% \times d = e$
Number non-farrowing sows detected as returns	114	96	190	$e \times b/100 = f$
Total pigs tested (non-returns)	886	904	810	$c - f = g$
Benefit of testing:				
Number of non-farrowing sows tested	6	24	10	$e - f = h$
Number of non-farrowing sows detected	5	22	9	$h \times \text{specificity}/100 = i$
Value of non-farrowing sows detected	£375	£1650	£675	$£75 \times i = j$
Number of false negatives	4	4	4	$(100-\text{sensitivity})(g - h) = k$
Cost of false negatives	£600	£600	£600	$k \times £150 = l$
Net benefit/loss per pig tested*	−25p	+116p	+9p	$(j - l)/g$

*From this must be deducted the cost of testing each pig plus an allowance for re-testing of negatives

Assumptions:
All sows not detected as returns are tested at 4 weeks after service.
80% of non-farrowing sows are in oestrus within 4 weeks of service.
Negative pigs are re-tested at 5 weeks then re-mated/culled by an average of 7 weeks after service.
In absence of test, empty sows not re-mated/culled until an average of 12 weeks after service and loss = £15 per week.
Financial benefit of acting on correct negative result = £75.
Accuracy of test = 99.5% on sows that farrow (sensitivity), 90% on non-farrowing sows (specificity).
Financial loss from culling and replacing false negative = £150.

test often show considerable variation in the accuracy attained. Of the many potential sources of error, those related to reproductive status are particularly important.

Pregnant pigs on one unit are much the same as on another, provided that similar stages of pregnancy are compared. Therefore data for the accuracy of a test on pigs which subsequently farrowed (the sensitivity) should be a good guide to the accuracy that can be expected in another herd testing at the *same time* after service. Any significant differences are likely to be due to competence, technique or equipment.

Non-farrowing pigs, however, are not such a homogeneous group. They may comprise pigs which return at a regular interval because pregnancy failed at an early stage, pigs with delayed returns and pigs with a variety of genital abnormalities (inactive ovaries, cystic ovaries, genital tract infections). They may also include pigs which were pregnant at the time of testing but whose pregnancy failed before farrowing. This means that accuracy on non-farrowing pigs (the specificity of a test) is very variable from one pig unit to another and even from one time period to another on the same unit. Predicting specificity requires knowledge of the reproductive condition of the non-farrowing pigs that will be tested and the effect this will have on the test contemplated. Alternatively the test can be evaluated *in situ*: comparing test results with subsequent farrowings, returns and abattoir examination of culls.

The important practical question regarding accuracy is "what is the probability that a positive pig will farrow and that a negative pig will not farrow"? These are known as the positive and negative predictive values of a diagnostic test and they vary from one pig unit to another, depending on what proportion of the pigs tested are going to farrow. This can be estimated from past experience in the herd. A lot of misleading information about pregnancy test accuracy stems from confusing predictive values with sensitivity and specificity.

Probability that positive

$$\text{pig will farrow (as \%)} = \frac{P \times F \times 100}{(P \times F) + (100-P)(100-N)}$$

Probability that negative

$$\text{pig will not farrow (as \%)} = \frac{N(100-P) - 100}{N(100-P) + P(100-F)}$$

where:

P = % of pigs tested that are likely to farrow
F = % accuracy of test when used on pigs that farrow (sensitivity)
N = % accuracy of test when used on pigs that do not farrow (specificity)

It can be seen from these formulae that the reliability of positive results will be higher in a herd where more of the pigs tested are truly pregnant (e.g. a herd with high fertility). On the other hand, more of the negative results will be errors, so culling negative pigs might be unwise.

DECIDING WHEN TO PREGNANCY TEST

The following points should be taken into account:

(1) The earlier empty sows are detected, the greater will be the economic benefit, *but* beware tests that promise an early result but whose negatives have to be confirmed by retesting or return to oestrus at a later date.
(2) Most pregnancy failures occur within 30 days of service, so testing *after* this time will produce less false positives in terms of predicting sows that will farrow.
(3) Some tests need to be undertaken at particular times after service for high accuracy. Others show improved accuracy with increasing time after service.
(4) If empty sows are to be re-mated, they should be tested shortly before the next anticipated return to oestrus, so that extra efforts can be made to detect it.

CONCLUSIONS

No pregnancy test emerges as clearly superior, so deciding which test to use becomes a matter of "horses for courses".

Achieving good results with any test (including non-return to oestrus) requires a certain amount of training and practice. A viable alternative to pregnancy testing may be to improve facilities and techniques for detecting returns to oestrus. None of the tests available at present is able to estimate litter size reliably in individual sows.

Real-time ultrasound and rectal palpation are highly accurate tests that can be used over a wide range of gestational stages but will not be appropriate for many situations on the grounds of cost and convenience.

The oestrone sulphate test has good accuracy, but sampling time is critical. A particularly good indication for it is the checking of pigs that do not appear to be "filling out" at about 12 weeks after service. The blood progesterone test has the advantage that it can be used to identify empty pigs before they return to heat, but accuracy will be poor if delayed returns are a problem. A-mode ultrasound can provide a cheap and simple pregnancy test, but tends to produce many errors. False negatives can be reduced by re-testing, but false positives will still reduce the potential benefit of testing.

When Doppler ultrasound is used to detect fetal sounds, false negatives are likely to be a problem. When Doppler instruments are used to detect uterine artery sounds there are likely to be less false negatives but occasional false positives. If negative pigs are re-tested to reduce errors, Doppler instruments emerge as superior to A-mode equipment. Re-testing does, however, increase the cost of testing and it increases the time before a final decision is made.

Quite often, when pregnancy-testing pigs, one class of results (positive or negative) must have minimal errors. For example, if selecting pregnant pigs for export, false positives are less acceptable than false negatives; whereas if culling negative pigs, false negatives will be less acceptable than false positives. In this context it is worth noting that the most reliable positives are produced by the Doppler (fetal sounds) and rectal palpation tests. The oestrone sulphate and real-time ultrasound tests can be added to these if there are not too many pregnancy failures after the time of testing. The most reliable negative results are achieved with the blood progesterone, non-return to oestrus, real-time ultrasound and rectal palpation tests. The oestrone sulphate test can be added to these if the time of sampling is precise.

Accuracy claims for pregnancy tests require careful appraisal because some methods of evaluation can be misleading. Similarly the economics of pregnancy testing are worthy of careful study in each practical situation. Whatever decision is made, it is advisable to undertake a periodic assessment of any routine testing that is undertaken in order to verify accuracy, check that results are being acted upon and confirm cost-effectiveness.

REFERENCES AND FURTHER READING

Almond, G. W. & Dial, G. D. (1986). Pregnancy diagnosis in swine: a comparison of the accuracies of mechanical and endocrine tests with return to oestrus. *Journal of the American Veterinary Medical Association* **189**, 1567.

Meredith, M. J. (1980). The Detection of Pregnancy in Pigs, Part 1: Tests for pregnancy. Tape-slide programme, Unit for Veterinary Continuing Education, Royal Veterinary College, London.

Meredith, M. J. (1981). The Detection of Pregnancy in Pigs, Part 2: Choosing a pregnancy test. Tape-slide programme, Unit for Veterinary Continuing Education, Royal Veterinary College, London.

CHAPTER 5

Induced Farrowing on Commercial Pig Farms

BILL MILLER

INTRODUCTION

Prostaglandins permit the synchronization of farrowing in groups of sows, so that as many as 90 % of farrowings can be reliably expected to occur on two working days of the week, and then mainly during normal working hours. In this way the producer can better allocate his labour resources, thereby improving perinatal care and largely avoiding farrowings at the weekends.

There have been many publications on the subject of induced farrowings with prostaglandins. However, until recently, nearly all the reports have been concerned with demonstrating that the various types of prostaglandin will induce parturition effectively and safely. Few studies demonstrate a positive benefit to the pig farmer. One reason for this is that utilization of the potential benefits of inducing farrowing are dependent upon management. Prostaglandins only allow the farmer an opportunity to exploit the benefits of controlled parturition.

METHODS OF USE

In view of the variation in gestation length between breeds
and between farms, the recommendation of use for prostaglandins has been linked to the pattern of farrowing on each
particular farm.

Sows and gilts are normally treated 1–2 days before the
expected date of farrowing, calculated from the average natural
gestation length for the herd. However, animals can be treated
as much as 3 days before term and provided that there is a
high standard of care during the perinatal period, this does
not cause any problems.

By injecting groups of sows at the appropriate stage of
gestation on Mondays and Thursdays, farrowings can largely
be restricted to 2 days in each week. However, some farmers
prefer to inject only those sows due at the weekend, plus
those which have not farrowed by Thursday of each week. In
this system, Friday becomes the main farrowing day.

In order to give the pig producer proper control over the
use of prostaglandin on the farm, he should be allowed to
administer the drug himself. However, prostaglandins are
highly potent and potentially dangerous compounds, and are
Prescription Only Medicines under the control of the veterinary profession. This does not mean that prostaglandins cannot
be safely administered by a responsible pigman and the
Veterinary Defence Society and the Pig Veterinary Society
have recently indicated that the correct way for a veterinarian
to approach this matter (should he or she wish to delegate
the job of injecting sows) is to have a nominated person on
the farm.

On farms where the spread of services is evenly distributed
throughout the week, it could be expected that 29 % of sows
would farrow during the weekend. However, this prediction
does not take into account the common management practice
of synchronized weaning on one working day of each week.

The day of weaning is usually chosen by the farmer so that
weaned sows will not come into oestrus during the weekend.
Wednesdays or Thursdays are common weaning days which
results in the majority of sows returning to oestrus on Tuesday
or Wednesday of the following week. Thus, if most of the
sows in each batch are served on Tuesday or Wednesday of

each week, by adding on 115 days, it can be seen that the majority of these sows will be due to farrow on Friday or Saturday, i.e. just at a time which is most inconvenient for the stockman. Paradoxically, by trying to make life easier for himself at one end of the breeding cycle, the stockman has made things more difficult at the other.

RESULTS

From Fig. 5.1, showing the pattern of farrowing on Farm 14 before and after the introduction of prostaglandin to control farrowing, it can be seen that there was a high proportion of sows farrowing late in the week and over the weekend (37% on Friday and Saturday; 30 % on Saturday and Sunday).

However, in 1979, selective induction of farrowing was

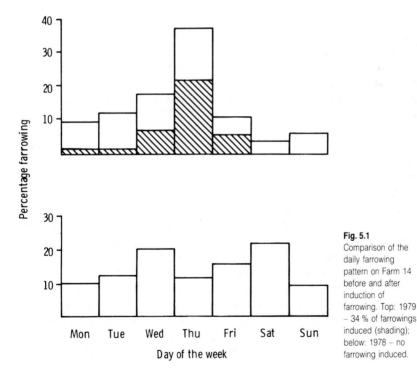

Fig. 5.1
Comparison of the daily farrowing pattern on Farm 14 before and after induction of farrowing. Top: 1979 – 34 % of farrowings induced (shading); below: 1978 – no farrowing induced.

introduced with around 34 % of sows being treated. This resulted in a peak of farrowings on Thursday of each week (38 %) and weekend farrowings were reduced to around 11 %.

Better results were obtained on Farm 3 (Fig. 5.2) where 74 % of all sows were treated with prostaglandin in 1981. This resulted in 53 % of all farrowings occurring on Friday of each week and weekend farrowings were reduced to 4 % .

Results from Farm 6 where 95 % of all sows were induced during 1982 are also shown (Fig. 5.3).The main farrowing day of each week was Tuesday with the rest of the activity confined to Thursday and weekend farrowings accounting for only 1 % of the total.

A comparison of gestation length distribution on Farm 6 before and after the use of prostaglandin (Fig. 5.4) shows that the mean gestation length of the herd in 1978, prior to the introduction of controlled farrowing, was 116.2 days. In 1981 this was reduced to 113.9 days, a mean difference of 2.3 days. Similar results were obtained on Farms 3 and 14 where the difference in mean gestation length pre- and post-induction of farrowing was 0.7 and 1.7 days respectively.

On Farm 6, prior to the introduction of induced farrowing, 82 % of sows were weaned on Wednesday of each week but there was still a "tail" of residual weanings throughout the rest of the week and into the weekend. However, following

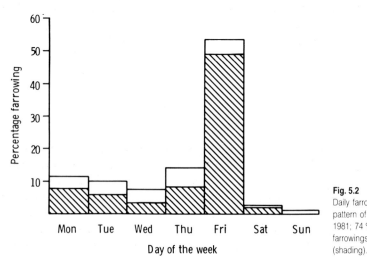

Fig. 5.2
Daily farrowing
pattern of Farm 3 in
1981; 74 % of
farrowings induced
(shading).

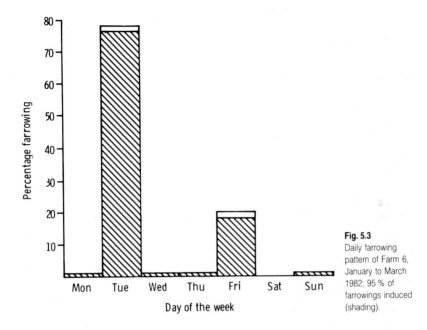

Fig. 5.3
Daily farrowing pattern of Farm 6, January to March 1982; 95 % of farrowings induced (shading).

the use of prostaglandin, all weaning was undertaken on 2 days of the week.

There was a trend towards lower numbers of stillbirths in the treated groups, although this was statistically non-significant.

Analysis of pre-weaning losses is not simple owing to the practice of interfostering (one of the benefits of synchronized farrowing). More piglets were fostered to and from treated sows on all farms.

DISCUSSION

The concentration of farrowing achieved by the use of prostaglandin on the farms illustrated gave the farmers considerable management benefits. Work-scheduling was made easier and supervision of farrowing was increased, although this may not have been exploited to its fullest extent. Although most modern pig farms still need cover at the weekends for feeding, etc., it is obviously a considerable advantage to avoid

Bill Miller

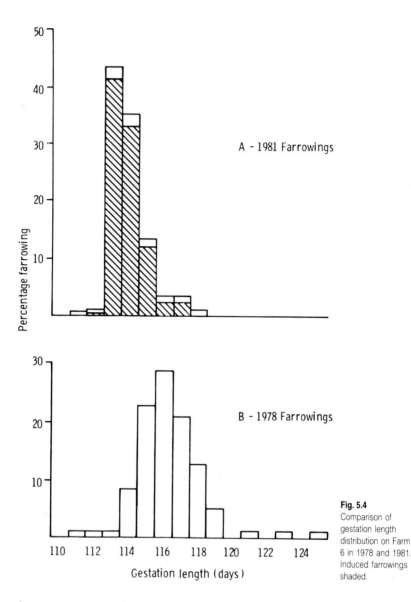

Fig. 5.4
Comparison of gestation length distribution on Farm 6 in 1978 and 1981. Induced farrowings shaded.

farrowings at weekends and during the night-time. The convenience of controlled farrowing has often been dismissed merely as an additional benefit. However, it is now apparent that employees demand, and will continue to demand, more organized and predictable work-schedules with planned leisure time. Furthermore, a reduction in the number of weekend and night-time farrowings should result in less overtime payments.

The ability to synchronize farrowing fits in well with modern pig management concepts and enables the farmer to feel that he has better control of the operation. Concentration of farrowings such as that achieved on Farm 6 offers excellent opportunities for interfostering of piglets at the right time (within 24 h of birth) and ensures that each piglet gets the right quantity and quality of colostrum at the right time.

With so many sows farrowing simultaneously, the opportunities for re-distributing piglets into litters of equal number and equal size are increased. As a result many piglets which would hitherto have been classified as "runts" can be gathered together in one or more litters in the care of a younger sow. Work by English (1976) has shown that litters containing piglets of uniform body size have better survival rates than those where the piglets are of unequal size.

The practice of interfostering makes interpretation of pre-weaning losses difficult. Consequently, the benefits resulting from improved perinatal care are more speculative. It appears that on those farms where the opportunities presented by prostaglandins have been properly exploited, an increase of up to 0.6 pigs weaned per litter, is possible. This appears to stem from reduced "stillbirths" (pigs that actually died immediately post-partum) and reduced pre-weaning mortality (probably arising from the more effective use of colostrum).

In the face of an apparent stillbirths problem on a farm, the institution of a controlled farrowing regime can be a useful form of therapy. Similarly, during periods when unusually large litters cause a shortage of available teats, it can be useful to induce one or more gilts to farrow and provide more interfostering opportunities. Such a system of "elective fostering" can also be useful in the case where it is desirable to farrow a sow unlikely to survive after farrowing (for example an imminent prolapse), alongside other normal sows.

The reduction in mean gestation length observed on all farms following the use of controlled farrowing is a significant benefit to the farmer if the management system is flexible enough to move forward the traditional weaning practice to take advantage of the extra days saved. If this is not possible, then the main effect will be to ·increase the average age of

Table 5.1 Potential financial benefits from prostaglandin-induced farrowings

	Gestation	Age at weaning*	Weaning to effective service* or culling	Farrowing index	Farrowings with 250 sows	Pigs weaned @ 9.2/litter	@ 9.5/litter
Not induced (1979)	116.2	23	14	2.38	596	5483	—
90 % induced (1981)	113.9	23	14	2.42	605	5566	5748
						(83 extra)	(265 extra)

*Fixed for this example.
With value of a weaned pig @ £20
Less creep feed @ £400/tonne 50p/weaner
Net value of an extra weaned pig £19.50
Cost of treatment/sow @ £1.15 × 90% × 250 × 2.42 = £626
Return to 83 extra pigs = £1619 (from shorter gestation)
        182 extra pigs = £3549 (from reduced pre-weaning mortality)
   Total 265 extra pigs = £5168

piglets at weaning. A reduction of 2.3 days in the mean gestation length and pre-losses reduced by 0.3 pigs per litter can be interpreted as an annual saving of around £5168 on a 250 sow herd (Table 5.1). This represents a significant improvement in the profitability of the enterprise since the extra pigs reared are "marginal pigs" which should not significantly increase any of the existing overheads of the business.

The concentration of weaning achieved on Farm 6 following the use of prostaglandin is a small but nevertheless important benefit to the farmer in the overall planning and organization of work schedules leading to greater efficiency and improved labour relations.

In conclusion, the use of prostaglandin to control farrowing has become an established routine on the three farms mentioned in this paper and now forms an integral part of their management policies. It is apparent, however, that the benefits of induced farrowing can only be achieved by exploitation of the opportunities offered by controlling the time of parturition.

FURTHER READING

English, P. R. (1976). *Proceedings of the Pig Veterinary Society* **1**, 105.
Miller, W. M. (1981). *In Practice* **3**, 16.

CHAPTER 6

Post Parturient Problems in Swine

JOHN CARR

DISORDERS OF THE MAMMARY GLANDS

Mammary disorders account for up to 50 % of the preweaning piglet losses on many farms. Sows need at least 12 functioning teats at parturition to raise an average litter of 10–11 piglets.

Each teat is supplied with milk from two or, occasionally, three mammary glands and this can lead to a problem in diagnosis of disease, as the milk that is expressed from the nipple may have originated from only one of the glands, the other gland being non-productive or diseased. Records of the sow mammary gland function should be kept on charts as shown in Fig. 6.1.

In the normal sow milk can be expressed in the immediate pre- and post-farrowing period. However, if difficulty is experienced, an intramuscular injection of 5 iu of oxytocin should result in milk flow in 10–15 min.

AGALACTIA

Usually the first clinical sign observed by the stockman is a litter of noisy, hungry, restless piglets which may appear gaunt and make frequent nursing attempts.

Teat	Left	Right
1		
2		
3		
4		
5		
6		
7		
Place an X for a nonfunctioning gland		

Fig. 6.1
Recording chart for mammary function.

Agalactia of the gilt

Bright, alert

The gilt has full painful mammary glands but does not produce any milk because of failure of milk let down. One intramuscular injection of 10 iu oxytocin may solve the problem.

Hyperexcitable – psychogenic agalactia

The gilt appears excited, restless, will not allow the piglets to suck, and will not call her piglets. She may react aggressively towards the piglets. There is no milk let down but the glands are full. Treatment with a sedative such as azaperone and the administration of 5 iu oxytocin intramuscularly usually resolves the situation. Taking the gilt for a walk may also help to ease the situation.

Coliform mastitis (Fig. 6.2)

The sow is depressed, inappetent and shows little interest in her piglets. Pyrexia is common (40.5–42°C). (The rectal temperature of healthy sows rises at parturition from the dry sow level of 38.7°C to 40°C 24 h after parturition. It then drops to 39.3°C for the remainder of the lactation period.) The clinical signs of coliform mastitis closely resemble *Escherichia coli* toxic mastitis of cattle.

Palpation of the sow's udder may reveal painful swollen oedematous glands. Blotchy reddening may be seen over the affected gland(s). Note that although glands may appear palpably normal, histologically they may show signs of change. The piglets often have diarrhoea.

Milk from the affected gland may be serous, purulent or blood stained. The cell count rises to 200×10^6/ml and the proportion of leucocytes in the sample may reach 75 %. This can easily be seen by taking a slide smeared with the milk and air dried. Stain with methylene blue for 30 s and examine under the microscope.

Milk for bacteriology needs to be taken as aseptically as possible and the results viewed critically as the causal agents are also normal environmental organisms, for example *E. coli* or *Klebsiella* species.

Vaccination for mastitis is often unsuccessful as a wide variety of *E. coli* serotypes have been found, often differing from one gland to another, in the same animal. *Klebsiella* species have been isolated and are often associated with sawdust bedding.

Non-affected glands often show agalactia for no apparent cause; however, recent work on the pathogenesis of this disorder has shown that *E. coli* endotoxin can produce a profound depression of prolactin levels for several hours after administration, which may explain this phenomenon.

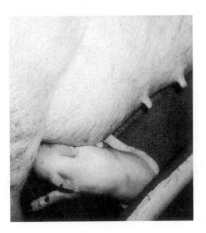

Fig. 6.2
A sow with an acute mastitis in a hind gland 24 h after farrowing.

Treatment

Acutely ill sows can be saved by parenteral treatment with antibiotics. An intramuscular injection of 5 iu of oxytocin will stimulate milk flow. Flunixin meglumine (Finadyne), two injections of 2 mg/kg intravenously 12 h apart, can be a life saver. The sow settles down within 4 h and is often suckling within 24 h. Offering the sow fresh food such as grass may help to stimulate an appetite.

Intravenous injection in the sow is often regarded as being very difficult. However, with patience and a steady hand an injection into one of the larger ear veins, particularly on the caudal aspect using a 18 gauge 1–1.5 in needle, will enable up to 20 ml to be administered reasonably easily.

In the more severely affected cases the prognosis is very poor but rehydration with saline given intravenously by a long catheter into the jugular vein and a flutter valve can give dramatic improvements in moribund animals. A sick sow will require approximately 7 l of saline to make any real difference to her state, but when they are this ill it is a matter of humane destruction or intensive therapy.

In many cases of coliform mastitis, the sow may be quite sick but rarely dies. Intensive therapy is required to restore milk supply and minimize permanent damage to the mammary glands.

Control

Methods of control are as follows:

   Improve the sows' farrowing environment.
   Ensure proper teeth clipping.
   Have adequate fly control.
   Healthy, fit, properly fed sows.
   Good effective management.

Non-infected agalactia

The affected animal appears similar to a sow suffering from coliform mastitis, but all milk expressed appears normal and the animal is only mildly pyrexic at 39.5°C. Neither mastitis nor metritis can be found.

Histologically the glands often resemble those of a sow at 110 days gestation. Very careful examination of the sow is needed to eliminate other causes of agalactia.

Hormonal causes have been suggested. Any imbalance in management or nutrition appears to predispose to the condition. This syndrome can severely affect a high proportion of farrowing sows in some herds at some time.

Treatment

The condition will resolve spontaneously after 3 days but by this time the litter may be lost. Treatment to save the litter is paramount. Administration of regular doses of 5–10 iu of oxytocin every 3 h has been shown to be beneficial. The use of one of the long-acting oxytocin products now under trial may be useful.

Flunixin meglumine has been shown to be very useful even when administered at 2.2 mg/kg intramuscularly. Many of these animals are constipated and the feeding of bran in the last week of pregnancy may help.

Lactation failure in the sick sow

Various causes of lactation failure are summarized in Table 6.1.

Nutritional factors affecting milk supply

Ergot poisoning

Chronic ergot poisoning (Fig. 6.3) causes agalactia in sows due to poor mammary gland development. The administration of oxytocin has no effect. The piglets are usually born small and they suffer heavy mortality because of their weak nature and lack of milk supply. There is no specific treatment. Removal of the contaminated ration should restore milk production.

Table 6.1 Lactation failure in the sick sow

Acute coliform mastitis	Pyrexic, inappetent, abnormal milk
Non-infected agalactia	Slight pyrexia, inappetent, normal milk
Metritis	Purulent foul smelling vulval discharge, pyrexic and inappetent
Acute eperythrozoonosis	Pyrexic and inappetent
	Mammary and vulval oedema
	Piglets pyrexic, may be anaemic and have jaundice
	Transmission by needles and teeth clipping equipment is possible
Undue stress	Sows require a room temperature of about 18°C
Heat stress	Piglets require a creep temperature above 30°C
Porcine stress syndrome	
Any other causes of systemic illness, e.g. erysipelas and transmissible gastroenteritis	

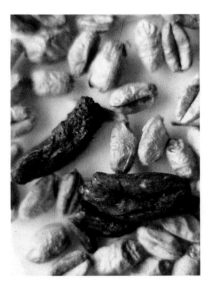

Fig. 6.3
Wheat heavily contaminated with ergot.

Water deprivation

There should be no minimum requirement, water should available at all times day and night. Ensure that the sow knows how to operate the drinker.

Examination of the mammary glands of the sow deprived of water will reveal several non-functional, dry glands and a few half-empty glands (Fig. 6.4). This is particularly evident at 2 weeks after farrowing when the milk production should be at its peak. Examination of the piglets will show uneven litters. Several of the sows may have a chalky discharge from their vulva caused by phosphate crystallization from the urine.

TEAT DAMAGE OR LOSS

Sows can suffer quite severe cuts to their teats (Fig. 6.5). Damage to teats affects suckling as the sow attempts to suckle but leaps up in pain, suddenly grunting and snapping at her piglets. The piglets' sharp teeth often exacerbate the condition by biting the nipple to hold on when the sow rises, causing more damage and pain to the sow.

Sows on floors that are slippery can also damage their teats,

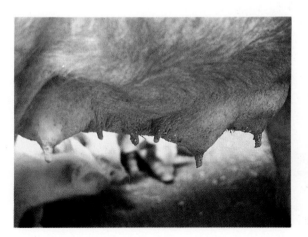

Fig. 6.4
Sow suffering from water deprivation. The middle three glands are dry.

particularly the rear three pairs, by standing on them as they get up or lie down.

Causes of non-functional teats

Table 6.2 summarizes the causes of non-functional teats.

DISORDERS OF THE GENITAL TRACT

ENDOMETRITIS AND METRITIS (Fig. 6.6)

A vulval discharge is normal in the healthy sow for up to 5 days after farrowing. This discharge can be variable in colour and consistency ranging from clear with yellow or blood specks to thick bloody material. The sow, however, is not sick or pyrexic. This "normal" discharge led to the misconception that mastitis, metritis and agalactia always occur as one syndrome.

The incidence of endometritis varies from 2 % to over 30 % on some farms often as a direct result of managemental factors.

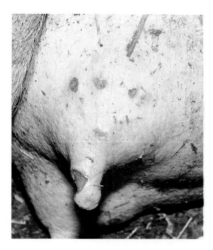

Fig. 6.5
Severe damage to a nipple.

Table 6.2 Reasons for non-functional teats

Hereditary defects	Blind teats
	Inverted nipples
	Poor mammary development
Nipple damage	Nipple necrosis from floor abrasion in first week of life
	Trauma from sow's feet
	Damage by piglets' teeth
Poor mammary development	Ergot poisoning
	Insufficient water suppy
	Deficient energy intake
Acute and chronic mastitis	Bacteria

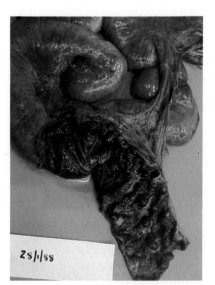

2s/ı/ss

Fig. 6.6
Severe bacterial metritis showing pus in the cervix and body of the uterus.

Bacterial endometritis

Environmental opportunist organisms are often responsible for bacterial endometritis in the United Kingdom.

Clinical signs

The sow has a purulent vulval discharge, is inappetent, lethargic and often pyrexic. She may have some degree of agalactia. The animal needs to be thoroughly examined including a vaginal and a rectal examination, which is not resented by most sows, but is difficult in gilts. Laceration of the vulva may be the cause of "vulval" discharges.

Treatment

Bacterial endometritis in most sows is mild and will resolve spontaneously. However, severe cases need parenteral antibiotics. The use of uterine irrigation is probably of little use considering the very large volume of the uterus at parturition. The uterus remains highly sensitive to oxytocin for several days after farrowing. However, once the piglets start sucking, the production of endogenous oxytocin will probably be enough to maintain uterine motility and involution. Animals which suffer any serious degree of endometritis should be culled as their future economic breeding prospects are doubtful.

Control

The sow and the farrowing quarters should be very clean. The stockman needs to observe good hygiene precautions. To avoid trauma of the genital tract the stockman must be very gentle, particularly in view of the modern trend towards 100 % manual intervention at all farrowing. If oxytocin is overused in cases of obstructive dystocia, uterine damage may result from spasms of the uterus.

Ensure faeces from behind the sow are removed manually in the period 3 days prepartum to 10 days postpartum. The sow often fails to clear faeces, even through well-designed slats, during this period as it is more sedentary. This will reduce contamination of the genital and urinary tract by faecal microorganisms.

RETAINED PLACENTA

The fetal membranes are often passed with each piglet or as a group up to 4 h after farrowing. If not passed within 24 h, a severe and often fatal metritis develops. Immediate removal and treatment with oxytocin and parenteral antibiotics is recommended (Fig. 6.7).

RETAINED FETUS

Retained fetus is difficult to diagnose (Fig. 6.8). The sow is still straining 24 h after farrowing. A piglet may be felt on rectal or vaginal examination. Note that ossified hypertrophic metaplasia of the mesentery can feel like a fetus. A B-mode real time ultrasound scanner with a 3.5 MHz transducer will visualize these piglets and can assist in making the diagnosis.

VAGINAL INJURIES

Vaginal injuries can be caused by:

Trauma from an obstructed piglet.
Rough handling by the stockman during an assisted far-

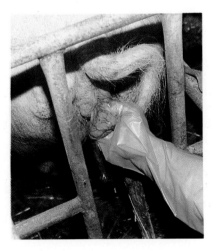

Fig. 6.7
Retained placenta being removed from a sow 36 h after farrowing.

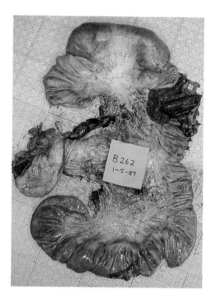

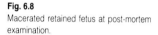

Fig. 6.8
Macerated retained fetus at post-mortem
examination.

rowing (Fig. 6.9). The piglet's feet are normally covered by
small collagen caps (thimbles or slippers) to protect the
uterus and vagina.
Biting from other sows.
Prolapse of the bladder can occur through the vaginal tear.

PROLAPSES OF THE GENITAL TRACT

Uterine prolapse

This occurs immediately after farrowing and the sow will
rapidly go into a severe state of shock. Fortunately this
condition is not common. Replacement should only be considered if the uterus is undamaged and the sow is fit
enough for anaesthesia. In many cases humane destruction, or
amputation followed by casualty slaughter, may be the only
option. Culling the sow may be necessary in the long term,
which makes surgery difficult to justify from an economic
aspect.

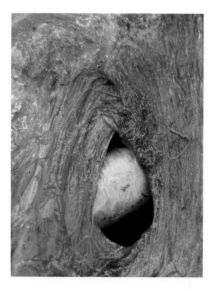

Fig. 6.9
Vaginal tear from a finger puncture.

Vaginal prolapse

A bulging mass is seen protruding from the vulva. It is more common in late pregnancy but can occur after farrowing. Treatment is by replacement of the prolapse and by placing a purse string suture around the vulva. Antibiotic cover may help to relieve the bacterial irritation. A rectal prolapse can also accompany a vaginal prolapse in sows. Prolapse may occur because the slope of the sow stall is too great. There is probably an hereditary predisposition to vaginal prolapses and so the sow should be used only as a terminal dam.

Retroposition of the bladder

Retroposition of the bladder may cause abdominal straining and therefore may complicate the diagnosis of a prolapse of vagina or rectum. The bladder (which may be an obstruction to replacing the vaginal prolapse) can be emptied by means of a flexible catheter, when it will assume a normal position.

SWOLLEN VULVA

A unilateral or bilateral enlargement of one lip of the vulva can be caused by traumatic injury at farrowing, by other sows biting the vulva, or from the rear stall gate, resulting in oedema or a haematoma. Treatment involves cleaning the vulva and applying petroleum jelly to prevent drying and cracking.

Bilateral enlargement is seen with zearalenone toxicity and signs can be produced by levels of 5 ppm in the diet. Oedema can also occur secondarily to eperythrozoonosis.

OTHER CONDITIONS OF THE POST PARTURIENT PERIOD

THE "DOWNER SOW"

The "downer sow" is not uncommon in the immediate postparturient period.

Lactation osteoporosis may make the bones weaker and more likely to fracture. This is exacerbated by poorly designed farrowing crates. Pelvic fractures lead to a sow adopting the posture shown in Fig. 6.10. There is no economic therapy in most cases. Calcium and phosphorus levels in the diet should be examined to reduce incidence of lactation osteoporosis.

Muscular weakness causes unsteadiness. These animals must be made to rise several times daily. Ideally, encourage exercise by allowing them out of the stall for 10 min twice daily. Analgesics such as phenylbutazone help to relieve any pain the sow is experiencing.

From the welfare aspect where the sow has trouble rising, moving her to a straw yard is to be recommended. If this is not possible, straw or a rubber pad should be placed under the sow to give her more grip. This will help to minimize the risk of pressure sores. Overgrown toes should be trimmed. Hypocalcaemia must be a differential diagnosis (see below).

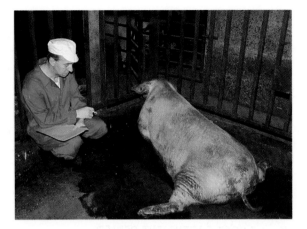

Fig. 6.10
Fractured pelvis after
farrowing.

HYPOCALCAEMIA

Hypocalcaemia in sows may go unrecognized. The clinical
signs following farrowing are restlessness and incoordination
followed by recumbency, coma and death. Response to treatment with 20 % calcium borogluconate by intravenous or
subcutaneous is rapid.

Subclinical cases could be suspected in farms with higher
than normal incidence of stillbirths, (due to protracted
farrowings), uterine inertia or retained afterbirth. Raising the
calcium level in the feed, if low, may help. In lactating sows
6 weeks after farrowing an eclampsic form may occur. Normal
blood levels of calcium average 2.7 mmol/l. Cases of hypocalcaemia have blood calcium levels of around 2 mmol/l.

CLOSTRIDIUM NOVYI

A sow which dies suddenly and the carcass starts decomposing
within hours of death with gross abdominal distension may
have been infected by *C. novyi*. The disease may also be seen
in the live animal where the sow is depressed at the start of
farrowing and develops uterine inertia. Upon examination
she is toxaemic, and moans in pain on vaginal or rectal
examination. A slight to moderate bloat is also seen. On

paracentesis gas is expelled from the peritoneal cavity. Rapid death often ensues.

The characteristic pathological sign is "Aero chocolate" liver. Definitive diagnosis can be made by fluorescent antibody examination of an impression smear made from infected liver tissue.

The pathogenesis of this disease is poorly understood. Vaccination with sheep clostridial vaccines has been advocated, but does not provide cover in all cases. The author has seen this condition more often associated with overweight sows. Reducing the bodyweight of sows has reduced the prevalence of the condition on certain farms.

PYELONEPHRITIS/CYSTITIS

Cases of pyelonephritis/cystitis seen in the farrowing house have chronic active pyelonephritis despite previously showing no clinical signs. The sow usually presents with a bloody vulval discharge, which is associated with haematuria and pyuria. The sow is inappetent and as the disease progresses the animal becomes more depressed and dies.

Many cases are associated with water deprivation. It is essential that the water supply in the farrowing house is adequate, that the drinkers operate with a flow rate of 2 l/min of fresh clean water, without too much water pressure, which would result in excessive water spillage. In many cases the water deprivation has resulted directly from a leaking water/feed trough or indirectly through the water/feed trough being filled with food, which soaks up all the available water. This is a particular problem as sows normally become inappetent at farrowing.

Treatment of individual sows can be attempted by administering water and encouraging the sow to urinate and by giving the sow exercise, ideally placing her in a straw yard with a creep area for the piglets. Antimicrobial therapy for 3 days using intramuscular injections of 100 mg lincomycin and 7.0 mg amoxycillin per 20 kg bodyweight has proved successful. The sow should be culled after weaning, as chronic renal changes cannot be resolved.

Disease

CHAPTER 7

Scours in Pigs

DAVID TAYLOR

INTRODUCTION

Scours occur in pigs of any age. A wide variety of aetiological agents is involved, several of which may be present in the animal at the same time. Some of these agents produce distinctive clinical signs or affect particular parts of the intestinal tract and infection with them can be readily identified on the farm. Others produce similar clinical signs which may only be distinguished by post-mortem examination, differential response to treatment or laboratory examinations.

"Scouring" is the passage of faeces containing excessive water which are therefore soft or fluid in consistency. It may be the result of excessive production of fluid, as in enterotoxic *Escherichia coli* diarrhoea, or caused by failure of the large intestinal epithelium to resorb normal quantities of fluid passing down the gut. The diarrhoea seen is, therefore, a product of complex processes in the intestine.

The tremendous ability of the colon to absorb fluid means that disease can occur in much of the small intestine and anterior larger intestine without causing diarrhoea. "Scours" are therefore only a partial guide to the occurrence of enteric disease and may also be so transient that they are not recorded by the average stockman.

This article concerns the differentiation of scours alone in the context of the problem, as seen by the veterinarian when called to the farm, i.e. clinical signs, post-mortem findings and the results of laboratory examinations.

HISTORY

The initial notification of the problem usually provides some sort of history. Before proceeding with a visit it is helpful to obtain details of the age of the animals affected, the number involved, the clinical signs noted, their duration and the presence or absence of mortality. This last detail is of particular relevance as on-farm post-mortem examinations can often allow a diagnosis to be made which cannot be obtained by study of the clinical signs alone, and it is useful to be prepared for this. It is also helpful to ascertain whether the pigs concerned have been recently purchased and their location on the farm. The nature of the diet, the antimicrobials present in the ration and a history of previous successful or unsuccessful treatment may also be of use.

Many of these facts may be determined after arrival on the farm but knowledge of them before arrival is helpful. They may allow a tentative diagnosis to be made and sufficient therapeutic agent to be taken to the farm for immediate use.

CLINICAL SIGNS

Clinical signs are so commonly related to age that the differentiation of diarrhoeas will be considered here on an age basis (Fig. 7.1). It is, however, possible for agents which normally occur in a particular age group in a partially immune herd to occur in pigs of virtually any age in a non-immune herd.

An affected group of pigs should be watched before active examination. The temperature of the accommodation, the behaviour of the pigs and the pattern of defecation may all be observed better from a distance. Even in pens with fully slatted floors, diarrhoea may be seen at the corners, on

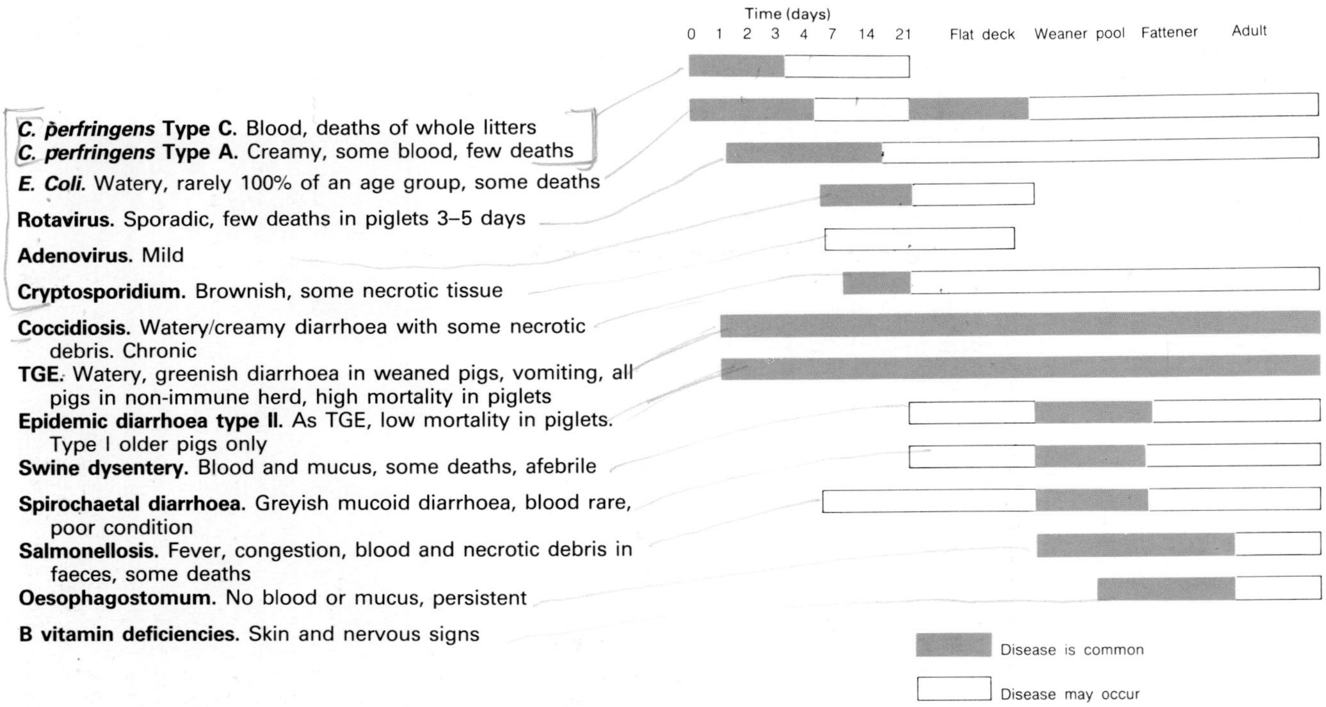

Time (days)

0 1 2 3 4 7 14 21 Flat deck Weaner pool Fattener Adult

C. perfringens Type C. Blood, deaths of whole litters
C. perfringens Type A. Creamy, some blood, few deaths

E. Coli. Watery, rarely 100% of an age group, some deaths

Rotavirus. Sporadic, few deaths in piglets 3–5 days

Adenovirus. Mild

Cryptosporidium. Brownish, some necrotic tissue

Coccidiosis. Watery/creamy diarrhoea with some necrotic debris. Chronic

TGE. Watery, greenish diarrhoea in weaned pigs, vomiting, all pigs in non-immune herd, high mortality in piglets

Epidemic diarrhoea type II. As TGE, low mortality in piglets. Type I older pigs only

Swine dysentery. Blood and mucus, some deaths, afebrile

Spirochaetal diarrhoea. Greyish mucoid diarrhoea, blood rare, poor condition

Salmonellosis. Fever, congestion, blood and necrotic debris in faeces, some deaths

Oesophagostomum. No blood or mucus, persistent

B vitamin deficiencies. Skin and nervous signs

Disease is common

Disease may occur

Fig. 7.1 Summary of clinical signs of diarrhoea in terms of onset and likely age of occurrence.

projections and, when undisturbed, on the slats themselves. Animals may be seen to defecate and this may be helpful.

The condition of the animal may also be a guide to the presence of disease. Pigs affected with swine dysentery are conspicuous by their sunken flanks. Dehydration may also be seen as may the congestive changes seen in classical salmonellosis. Faecal staining of the perineum may occur – clear faeces in neonatal *E. coli* (Fig. 7.2) but pasting in red or cream for the clostridial infections. The colour of the faeces may be a guide to diagnosis – the claret-coloured faeces of a typical *Clostridium perfringens* type C infection and the blood in faeces from animals infected with *C. perfringens* type A and swine dysentery, are all of diagnostic significance (Figs 7.3 and 7.4).

Mucus and necrotic material may also be relevant. They may be seen more clearly in individual undisturbed motions in rectal faecal samples or after suspension in water when mucus is the last to settle. Upon capture, affected pigs may pass faeces or a rectal sample may be taken. Many diarrhoeic pigs have empty rectums and repeated massage may be necessary to obtain faeces. Rectal temperatures should also be taken as they may be raised in cases of salmonellosis.

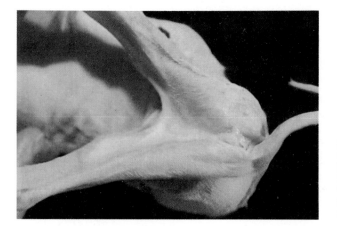

Fig. 7.2
Escherichia coli
infection. Perineum of
dehydrated piglet.
Watery faeces may
be seen only with
difficulty.

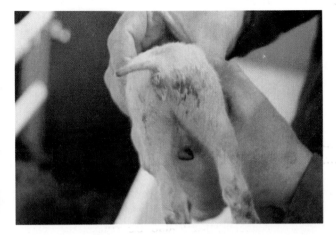

Fig. 7.3
Clostridium perfringens type A infection. Thin, live piglet with pasting of perineum.

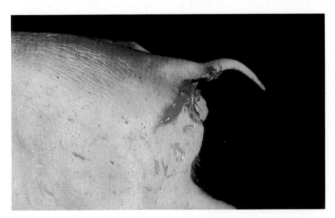

Fig. 7.4
Carcass of piglet infected with *Clostridium perfringens* type C, with typical pasting of red diarrhoea over the perineal region.

DIARRHOEA IN ALL PIGS IN A HERD

Two major diseases can present in this way. They are transmissible gastroenteritis (TGE) and epidemic diarrhoea. In classic outbreaks of TGE in non-immune herds, animals of all ages are often affected. As the disease is often transmitted by starlings or recently purchased animals, outbreaks may originate in sows or other pigs in open runs or buildings exposed to birds. Many outbreaks occur in the winter months but this is not exclusively the case. Furthermore, none have yet been reported from Scotland so herd location is a point of differentiation.

TGE is characterized by an explosive outbreak of diarrhoea, which is greyish or greenish in adults and greyish or yellowish in younger pigs and which spreads through the herd. It is often accompanied by vomiting and sows may abort. In classic TGE there is considerable mortality in neonatal pigs, but where drinkers are made available to piglets as routine this may be much reduced, especially when electrolytes are also routinely available.

In epidemic diarrhoea, a similar syndrome may be seen. Mortality may be lower in the neonatal piglets which may be unaffected in some patterns of the disease, but now that infection can be identified by serological means, it has become clear that mortality can occur in outbreaks of this condition. A presumptive diagnosis of TGE can, however, be made on these clinical signs but the disease in individual age groups will be considered below.

DIARRHOEA IN SUCKING PIGS

The aetiological agents of the diarrhoeic diseases of sucking pigs have incubation periods which allow a certain differentiation of the conditions according to the age at which they first appear. In some cases the disease may recur from that time on in non-immune piglets in an altered form or in combination with other enteric infections. Massive infections may move the age of onset forward. Unsatisfactory conditions of husbandry such as poor colostral uptake, chilling, agalactia among sows and poor hygiene may increase the morbidity and mortality rates in this age group in particular.

6–24 h old

First to appear (6–24 h of age) are bacterial infections caused by *E. coli*, *C. perfringens* and, possibly, campylobacters and streptococci. Neonatal *E. coli* diarrhoea is watery, profuse and often pale and yellowish in colour (Fig. 7.2). Piglets rapidly become dehyrated, lose condition, become depressed and may stand around with drooping tails and erect coat hairs, eventually dying in convulsions. The diarrhoea may dry rapidly under creep lamps and may only be seen as yellowish crusts on the perineum and thighs of affected piglets. When a thermometer or swab is inserted into the rectum, the diarrhoea oozes out. It is rare for more than 70 % of the litter to be affected by this condition. A history of vaccination of the sows, feedback or the correct use of genetically resistant stock may reduce the possibility that such a diarrhoea is caused by *E. coli*.

Neonatal *E. coli* diarrhoea may continue to appear until 3–4 days of age, and *E. coli* may cause diarrhoea in piglets sucking non-immune mothers (often gilts) at any age. It may also complicate diarrhoea caused by other agents and may initiate a chronic diarrhoea from which the agent has largely disappeared. In these cases, younger pigs must be examined to confirm the part played by *E. coli* in the initiation of the syndrome.

24–48 h old

C. perfringens type C causes an unmistakable, claret-red diarrhoea which is usually fatal within 12–24 h following infection. It occurs, within 24–48 h of birth and often affects several complete litters. Animals passing the red diarrhoea usually die if untreated and piglets may die without the stockman being aware of the characteristic red faeces. Affected animals often appear dull and may have pasting of the reddish diarrhoea over the perineal region (Fig. 7.4). Rectal temperatures are often depressed and if no diarrhoea is visible in the pen, a thermometer or rectal swab will soon elicit some. These classic signs may not occur in piglets of more than 4 days of age. In recovering older piglets necrotic material may appear in the faeces and chronic diarrhoea and marked loss of condition may ensue. The agent may complicate infection with other agents such as TGE in older piglets and its presence and contribution to the syndrome can only be distinguished in these animals by response to treatment, post-mortem examination (Fig. 7.5) and laboratory means.

C. perfringens type A produces a similar but much milder syndrome in animals of a similar age group (Fig. 7.3). Affected piglets are depressed, have marked pasting of the perineum

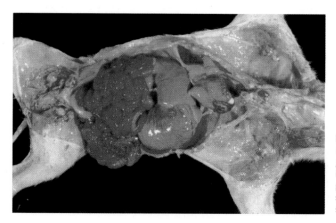

Fig. 7.5
*Clostridium
perfringens* type C
infection. Typical
post-mortem picture
showing inflamed
small intestine.

and pass a whitish diarrhoea often containing spots of blood
or with a pinkish tinge. Mortality is rare but recovering
animals may remain in poor condition for 3–5 days or longer.

Campylobacters may infect the neonate and in non-immune
animals may cause a creamy mucoid diarrhoea within the first
few days of life. After 48 h of age, however, they may be
responsible for the presence of mucus in diarrhoea of any
cause (Fig. 7.6)

Streptococci (especially *Streptococcus durans*) may also cause
a watery diarrhoea which is difficult to distinguish from *E.
coli* diarrhoea (Fig. 5.7).

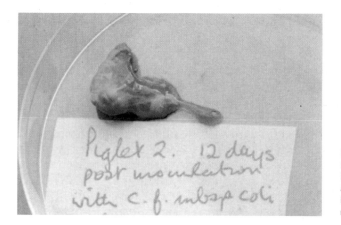

Fig. 7.6
Campylobacter coli
infection. Faeces
after experimental
infection. Note
mucus.

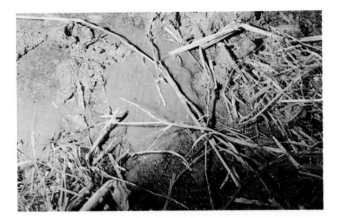

Fig. 7.7
Faeces from case of
spirochaetal
diarrhoea. Faint spots
of blood are present.

48 h onwards

From 48 h onward TGE, epidemic diarrhoea and rotavirus
infections may all occur. All cause a watery diarrhoea which is
difficult to distinguish solely on clinical grounds in individual
animals, but the diseases may be distinguished in the herd
as a whole.

In TGE, piglets may vomit milk curd and develop a watery
diarrhoea which may be greenish or grey, contain undigested
milk floccules and may sometimes be foul-smelling. Piglets in
the first week of life may be flushed and are often dehydrated
and covered with faeces. Faeces may be squirted at walls and
are passed in an effortless stream. After 2–3 days those piglets
surviving may develop complications caused by other agents
and only cases of recent onset should be examined. Death
from dehydration is common and mortality may reach 100 %
in piglets under 7 days of age in the absence of supplementary
fluid. The occurrence of vomiting, with disease in all age
groups, a history of TGE nearby and mortality in young
piglets, are signs indicative of TGE.

In epidemic diarrhoea the clinical signs may be similar but
mortality is less commonly seen and distinction between TGE
and epidemic diarrhoea can be made on this point. Once
again, in a non-immune herd, pigs of all ages may be affected.

Rotavirus infections are of short duration (3–5 days) usually
fail to result in mortality and only occasionally affect pigs of
other age groups. Some vomiting may occur 'and mortality

may reach 30 % in some litters and some outbreaks. This is, however, unusual and mortality is usually rare. They may occur at any stage through the sucking period but are common at 14 days of age. More than one antigenic type of rotavirus exists and rotavirus diarrhoea caused by a type to which there is no immunity may occur later in the pig's life.

Piglets recovering from any of these infections may pass pale or poorly-formed motions owing to failure to digest and absorb milk. All three diseases may occur in individual colostrum-deprived piglets in non-immune herds. Diarrhoea in these individuals cannot be distinguished without laboratory examination but a past history of the presence of appropriate agents may be of value.

72 h onwards

From 72 h onwards cryptosporidium may be able to initiate disease. A watery, sometimes brownish, diarrhoea may develop which contains shreds of necrotic material. Affected piglets are depressed, lose condition, may vomit and may die. Only in heavily contaminated farrowing accommodation would piglets of non-immune sows develop disease at this early stage as it is more common at about 10 days of age. Wet or sloppy faeces is likely to be passed for 3–5 days. Infection may also be inapparent.

96 h onwards

Coccidiosis and adenovirus infection, the last of the diarrhoeic conditions to appear, are first seen at 4–5 days of age. Adenovirus infection has an incubation period of 4–5 days in experimental conditions and is unlikely to occur in pigs younger than 5 days of age. The diarrhoea is mild, without blood or mucus, and occurs for 4–5 days only. Diagnosis on clinical grounds is difficult.

In coccidiosis a transient pasty diarrhoea or a profuse yellowish watery diarrhoea may occur to cause depression of growth, loss of condition and stunting. It may recur in successive litters, particularly in dirty conditions. As the diarrhoea becomes chronic it may contain some shreds of necrotic material and affected piglets may die.

These conditions have been dealt with according to the time of first onset but all (with the exception of the clostridial conditions) may initiate disease in older sucking piglets at a later age and several agents may occur at the same time. In addition, unchanged or stale creep feed may be associated with diarrhoea once creep feed has been supplied.

WEANED PIGS

The age of weaning varies between 2 and 8 weeks but is usually at 3–4 weeks in the UK. The dietary change may be the direct cause of diarrhoea, but in most cases the withdrawal of maternal antibody and mixing are more important. A change in antimicrobial content of the ration may also occur at this stage and husbandry factors such as chilling are also important. The most important feature of the diarrhoea seen in weaned and adult pigs is that the faeces are usually green, brown, blackish or greyish rather than white, as milk has been withdrawn from the ration. The basal composition of the diet of barley or maize may affect faecal colour. Diseases such as rotavirus infection, TGE, epidemic diarrhoea and *E. coli* infection therefore produce darker coloured diarrhoea in these older pigs than in sucking pigs.

E. coli diarrhoea occurs within 3–5 days after weaning or following dietary change, mixing of immune and non-immune pigs or withdrawal of an antimicrobial agent. Greyish or brownish watery diarrhoea with no traces of blood is passed by 20–50 % of all pigs in the batch. In flat decks or straw yards this faeces is sometimes difficult to detect and examination of the pen and especially dark corners near drinkers or at the edges of the mesh may be necessary. A torch is often helpful. Diarrhoeic faeces may be seen on the slurry crust after it has slipped through slat or mesh floors.

Affected pigs lose condition and become mildly fevered (to 40.5°C) and dehydrated. They often show little interest in food and may twitch their tails. Mortality is usually less than 10 % in this condition but the loss of condition may continue for some time.

E. coli is the most common of the post-weaning conditions and, unless animals have been vaccinated or are on an antigenic or antimicrobial ration, this is the condition from which others must be distinguished.

Another diarrhoea complex, which is rarely seen before eight to 14 days after weaning and mixing, is the swine dysentery/spirochaetal diarrhoea complex.

Swine dysentery is easily diagnosed in its classic form as the faeces of affected pigs contain blood, mucus and, occasionally in later cases, necrotic debris. No other syndrome in weaned pigs consistently contains this combination. The ammoniacal smell is also characteristic. Bloody, mucoid faeces are passed for 3–5 days after which they become mucoid, greyish or blackish and of soft consistency. Chronic diarrhoea may persist for days or weeks after the disappearance of clinical dysentery and contain varying amounts of mucus. Affected pigs are afebrile, lose gut fill and may become gaunt and dehydrated. They lose their appetite and lie in pen corners, but acute congestion of the ears is rarely seen.

Most pigs in a pen will eventually become affected. The spread of the disease is encouraged by mixing and a history of purchase 8–14 days previously may pinpoint the origin of the disease, which has an incubation period of 6–14 days or more. Up to 25 % of pigs may die in untreated outbreaks. The disease may occur in any age of pig other than sucking pigs in which it is only seen when the sow develops the disease. The clinical signs of swine dysentery can be affected by the presence of products such as dimetridazole, olaquindox or spiramycin in the ration.

Spirochaetal diarrhoea occurs within the same time limits but is more difficult to identify clinically or to separate from other syndromes. Affected pigs lose condition and pass a greyish mucoid diarrhoea. There is little blood and no necrotic material and deaths are rare. The spirochaetes concerned frequently complicate other syndromes and a primary diagnosis should not be reached on clinical signs alone. It may, however, be considered when a diarrhoea of this type is accompanied by poor growth rates.

Salmonellosis may occur at any age but *Salmonella choleraesuis* infections are not likely to occur in flat decks. At any time other salmonellae may cause a diarrhoea in which some blood or necrotic material may occur. This may be accompanied by fever (to 41.5°C) and some deaths. When diarrhoea of this type is seen in depressed pigs with cyanosis of the extremities and a tendency to huddle in straw (if available), salmonellosis should be considered possible and appropriate samples taken for laboratory confirmation. In the absence of fever, this diarrhoea may be distinguished from others by the presence of necrotic material and blood without mucus; however, these features are not always present and clinical signs alone cannot always be used to reach a diagnosis of salmonellosis.

Rotavirus may cause diarrhoea at any age when non-immune pigs are exposed to rotavirus or pararotavirus. Outbreaks are usually limited to small numbers of pigs which recover within 3–5 days after passing a brownish-grey diarrhoea. This infection cannot be diagnosed by clinical signs alone.

TGE and epidemic diarrhoea cause a similar syndrome. In the non-immune herd all weaned pigs or all those of 30 kg or over develop inappetence and a profuse watery, greyish green fetid diarrhoea or less dramatic greyish loose faeces which may be accompanied by vomiting. Vomiting is difficult to detect in a group of weaned pigs as the pale meal vomit is rapidly eaten by other pigs in the same group. No fever occurs and the disease lasts for 3–7 days in an individual group. Other factors may complicate recovery, e.g. dysentery and deaths from salt poisoning may occur in younger weaned pigs and those receiving liquid feed. Outbreaks of TGE may be distinguished from those of epidemic diarrhoea when mortality in young pigs is seen but in fattening units the two diseases are indistinguishable on clinical grounds. Individual cases or groups with either disease in herds where the diseases are enzootic cannot be diagnosed as such on clinical grounds.

Other diarrhoeas may occur in small groups of animals or following dietary change. A number of infectious agents could be involved and these include *Campylobacter jejuni* (some blood or mucus in a diarrhoea of short duration and no mortality), *Yersinia enterocolitica* (watery diarrhoea, short duration) and oesophagostomum infection. In some cases a dietary component may be involved but this is often difficult to confirm, although diarrhoeas have been described in vitamin B deficiencies such as riboflavin and nicotinamide deficiency (accompanied by skin changes) or pantothenate deficiency in which it may be accompanied by goose-stepping.

Scours in adults

Adults may be affected by salmonellosis, swine dysentery, spirochaetal diarrhoea, epidemic diarrhoea, TGE and, from time to time, by incidents of rotavirus or *E. coli* infection. They may also be infected by oesophagostomum and all these conditions may produce diarrhoeas resembling those seen in fattening animals on similar diets.

RESPONSE TO TREATMENT

Viral, coccidial, helminth and cryptosporidial infections will all be unaffected by antimicrobial treatment.

Clostridial infections will be reduced and eliminated by penicillins but not affected by neomycin and other aminoglycosides.

Penicillin will not affect *E. coli*, campylobacter, salmonella or the spirochaetal diseases (the latter are penicillin-sensitive but the drug rarely reaches the large intestine). Dimetridazole, ronidazole, tiamulin, organic arsenicals, spiramycin, tylosin and lincomycin are primarily active against swine dysentery and spirochaetal diarrhoea. They do not affect *E. coli* or salmonella infections but may reduce clostridial or campylobacter infections.

Semisynthetic penicillins, neomycin, spectinomycin, carbadox and sulphonamides, tetracyclines and chloramphenicol may be active against salmonellae and *E. coli*.

Amprolium, monensin and other anticoccidials may eliminate coccidia but monensin also has some action on swine dysentery.

These factors may be used to form an opinion about the identity of a diarrhoea. The patterns outlined above are complicated by resistance but are, nevertheless, of value in reaching a provisional clinical diagnosis.

POST-MORTEM FINDINGS

Gross post-mortem examinations can be carried out on the farm. The state of the pig carcass, the appearance of organs other than the gut and the regions of the gut to be affected may all be recorded. The gut can be examined in detail from the serosal surface, the appearance of its contents recorded and the appearance of the mucosa studied grossly and with a hand lens to record the height of the villi. Samples may be taken for laboratory confirmation. Post-mortem examinations will rarely be carried out on older animals with diseases such as TGE, epidemic diarrhoea, rotavirus or spirochaetal diarrhoea as deaths are rare in these age groups. Most pigs examined routinely will be young. This guide therefore takes account of the easily observable features. The most consistent of these are at gut level.

SMALL INTESTINAL DISEASE

Villous atrophy

Virus diseases such as TGE, epidemic diarrhoea and rotavirus cause villous atrophy but no necrosis, blood or inflammation will be present on the mucosa or in the gut contents. In chronic infections villous atrophy may be restricted to one part of the gut or complicated by secondary infection. In adenovirus infection only 20 % of the villi are shortened.

These conditions cannot be distinguished by post-mortem examination alone although gastric hyperaemia and ulceration may indicate TGE rather than the others. Laboratory diagnosis on live pigs is necessary to confirm.

Villous atrophy and inflammation

C. perfringens type C will cause total loss of villous structure and a claret-red gut will be seen (small and large intestine) in 2–4-day-old pigs, an unmistakable sign (Fig. 7.5). *C. perfringens* type A will cause villous atrophy, some necrosis, inflammation, pasting of hindlimbs and large intestinal involvement with some blood.

Villous atrophy and necrosis

Both cryptosporidium and, more commonly, coccidiosis may cause this in 10-day-old pigs. In cryptosporidial infection, changes are most common in the ileum and the serosal surface is uniform. In coccidiosis variable amounts of inflammation accompany the mucosal changes and the distended small intestine often appears spotted and grossly thickened, especially in the ileal region. There are no consistent large intestinal changes.

Salmonellosis may also cause this type of lesion but in most cases there will be some indication of systemic disease such as an enlarged spleen, petechiated kidneys and congested lymph nodes, especially of the mesenteric region: the large intestine will often be affected as well.

Little or no villous atrophy

Early *E. coli* diarrhoea causes gastric distension with milk or feed, a distended, thin walled, small intestine, often with watery contents and sometimes with flecks of yellowish milk (in piglets), and an empty colon. The intestinal mucosa is mildly hyperaemic and the villi are initially intact but may become shortened later. The remainder of the carcass is dehydrated but normal.

Other changes

Small intestinal proliferation of the mucosa and intestinal haemorrhage with blood clotting in the lumen, especially in the ileum, may be seen in weaned pigs with proliferative intestinal adenopathy. This condition does not cause diarrhoea *per se* but may underlie cases of apparent spirochaetal diarrhoea.

Blackened contents may result from gastric ulceration. The mucosa will be unaffected.

Ileal thickening with enlarged oedematous lymph nodes and mucoid ileal small and large intestinal contents may indicate the presence of *Campylobacter coli, C. jejuni* or *C. hyointestinalis* infection.

LARGE INTESTINAL DISEASES

Swine dysentery is the most common disease to be found post mortem. The large intestine is flaccid, may be reddened and contains mucoid, bloody contents. There may be bleeding points in the mucosa which is inflamed, thickened and may have necrotic debris on it. In more chronic cases the contents are khaki and contain mucus or necrotic debris; the mucosa may be lowered and free from necrotic debris. The remainder of the carcass is usually dehydrated and normal apart from an empty stomach, sometimes with gastritis.

In spirochaetal diarrhoea, changes are also restricted to the colon and involve mild inflammation of the wall with homogeneous, mucoid contents. As this condition is rarely fatal, it may be seen incidentally with diseases such as proliferative intestinal adenopathy or proliferative haemorrhagic enteropathy, which are fatal.

Oesophagostomum infections may also be seen as incidental findings. Worms may be seen on the colonic mucosa which is thickened and filled with pale nodules. The white nodules seen on the serosal surface in chronic colitis do not indicate this condition specifically; they are in fact inflamed lymphoid areas around crypts which penetrate the lamina propria.

LABORATORY FINDINGS

Samples taken from live animals or at post-mortem examination may be submitted to a laboratory for examination. Samples may include serum (preferably paired or at least from recovered pigs), faeces from untreated acutely affected pigs or tissue or gut taken post mortem. The faeces may be submitted whole, in saline or on swabs, preferably in transport medium. Organs for microbiological examination should be chilled and those for histology should be fixed.

The clinician may wish to request examination for a particular agent and a brief guide to the examinations possible is given in Table 7.1.

Table 7.1 Guide to examination for causal agents

Viral agents may be identified by:
  Electron microscopy of faecal suspension (rotavirus, para-rotavirus, adenovirus, calicivirus, astrovirus and, sometimes, coronavirus and enterovirus)
  Polyacrilamide gel electrophoresis (rotavirus and pararotavirus)
  Direct or indirect enzyme-linked immunosorbent assay (ELISA) tests on faeces (epidemic diarrhoea virus and rotavirus)
  Direct or indirect immunofluorescence on frozen tissues (TGE, epidemic diarrhoea)
  Virus isolation (TGE)
  Serum antibody demonstration (TGE, epidemic diarrhoea)
  Histology (adenovirus infection)

Bacterial agents may be demonstrated by:
  Direct smears of faeces or mucosa – clostridia, spirochaetes, vibrios (campylobacters) are all distinctive as are yeasts
  Direct or indirect immunofluorescence (*Treponema hyodysenteriae*)
  Identification of toxin in gut loops (*C. perfringens* type C, mouse protection test), in faeces *E. coli* cytotoxin, *C. perfringens* type A enterotoxin and α toxin.
  Isolation *E. coli*, *C. perfringens* type A, *T. hyodysenteriae*, spirochaetes of spirochaetal diarrhoea, campylobacters, *Yersinia enterocolitica*, salmonellae

Parasites may be demonstrated by:
  Flotation methods and wet smears of faeces – coccidia, cryptosporidia and *Oesophagostomum* species. Smears of faeces stained by modified acid-fast methods (cryptosporidia)
  Whole gut counting – (oesophagostomum)

Histological techniques are of value in adenoviral, cryptosporidial, coccidial and worm infections and the agents can be demonstrated. Material fixed in 10 % formol saline from freshly killed animals is of considerable value in confirming a clinical diagnosis or of revealing the presence of changes such as those of proliferative intestinal adenopathy which would otherwise go undiagnosed.

INTERPRETATION OF LABORATORY FINDINGS

A provisional diagnosis may be reached on clinical and pathological grounds on the farm and treatment and control measures initiated. If no diagnosis can be reached symptomatic treatments are often initiated.

The full laboratory report, which may arrive weeks later, must be interpreted with care by the clinician. A simple report saying that "β-haemolytic *E. coli* were present in the sucking pig faeces sample" may not be helpful. However, a report saying that "β-haemolytic K88 positive *E. coli* were isolated in pure culture in aerobic microaerophilic and anaerobic culture; virus particles were seen by direct electron microscopy or detected by ELISA tests for rotavirus or epidemic disease; no cryptosporidia or coccidia could be demonstrated; and the *E. coli* isolated was sensitive *in vitro* to antimicrobials A, B, and C", indicates that the *E. coli* is likely to have been the cause of the condition.

Remember, too, that the laboratory may have received unsatisfactory material, possibly delayed in the post and possibly from recovering or treated animals. They may have carried out only the examination requested; few laboratories investigate all samples for all possible agents. If appropriate control measures do not appear to be effective, the diagnosis originally reached should be reconsidered and additional information sought.

FURTHER READING

Adenovirus

Coussement, W., Ducatelle, R., Charlier, G. & Hoorens, J. (1981). *American Journal of Veterinary Research* **42**, 1905.
Sanford, S. E. & Hoover, D. M. (1983). *Canadian Journal of Comparative Medicine* **47**, 396.

Porcine epidemic diarrhoea

Bollwahn, W. (1983). *Pig News and Information* **4**, 141.
Coussement, W., Ducatelle, R., Debouck, P. & Hoorens, J. (1982). *Veterinary Pathology* **19**, 46.
Wood, E. N. (1977). *Veterinary Record* **100**, 243.

Transmissible gastroenteritis

Pritchard, G. C. (1982). *Veterinary Record* **110**, 465.
Wood, E. N. (1979). *British Veterinary Journal* **135**, 305.

Rotavirus

Bywater, R. J. & Woode, G. N. (1980). *Veterinary Record* **106**, 75.
Woode, G. N., Bridger, J. C., Hall, G. A., Jones, J. M. & Jackson, G. (1976). *Journal of Medical Microbiology* **9**, 203.

Salmonellosis

Linton, A. H. (1981). *Pig News and Information* **2**, 25.

Campylobacters

Taylor, D. J. & Olubunmi, P. A. (1981). *Veterinary Record* **109**, 112.

Swine dysentery

Alexander, T. J. L. & Taylor, D. J. (1969). *Veterinary Record* **85**, 59.
Lysons, R. J. & Lemcke, R. M. (1983). *Veterinary Record* **112**, 203.

Spirochaetal diarrhoea

Taylor, D. J., Simmons, J. R. & Laird, H. M. (1980). *Veterinary Record* **106**, 324.

Coccidiosis

Roberts, L., Walker, E. J., Snodgrass, D. R. & Angus, K. W. (1980). *Veterinary Record* **107**, 156.
Stuart, B. P., Lindsay, D. S. Ernst, J. V. & Gosser, H. S. (1980). *Veterinary Pathology* **17**, 84.

CHAPTER 8

Streptococcus suis type 2 in British Pig Herds

TERRY HEARD

INTRODUCTION

Various streptococci have been associated with clinical disease in pigs for some years. In the 1950s the British Veterinary Association's report on diseases of farm livestock described a clinical syndrome in which meningitis and/or arthritis caused by a streptococcus affected pigs between 2 and 6 weeks of age.

The earliest signs of infection were a raised temperature and anorexia. Affected animals displayed a swaying gait followed by an increasing inability to maintain balance, until they lay on their sides and made paddling movements with all four legs. Swollen joints were also noted and if the animal recovered, the swelling sometimes persisted for several months. This original summary of the condition is difficult to improve upon, although the syndrome described has taken on a far more obtrusive character in pig farms in the United Kingdom during the 1970s and 1980s.

It is now generally considered that the disease described in 1956 was not caused by a *Streptococcus suis* type 2, but rather by a type 1 version which was a singular capsule type, and it was not until 1973 that Windsor and Elliott reported the presence of type 2 in East Anglia. It is a matter for debate how long this subtype had been present in the British pig industry; it had certainly been recorded in Holland 10 years earlier (de Moor, 1963).

By 1974 outbreaks were being reported in numerous pig herds with the disease being characterized by sudden onset, mortality levels of between zero and 20 % and an age incidence of between 1 and 16 weeks. It appeared in a variety of husbandry and feeding systems, with symptoms of incoordination, collapse, paralysis and paddling of the limbs in a recumbent state. Death often followed. The sudden onset of the condition and its equally sudden disappearance make the assessment of treatment and preventive measures difficult.

PATHOGENESIS

Typically, the disease occurs in 6–8-week-old piglets; out of 50 piglets at risk two may die daily over a period of 3–5 days. Other cases, if treated and carefully nursed, can recover. As farm staff became more able to spot cases at an early stage, so recovery rates became greater.

Following such an episode the disease may "disappear" and not be recognized for a period, often 6 months or more, after which time it may suddenly reappear. It is this apparent unpredictability which has given rise to many of the claims for successful prevention and treatment that occur in the clinical clubs and groups in the pig industry.

DIAGNOSIS

Diagnosis of streptococcal meningitis is best obtained by isolating the organism by culture from the brain and confirming its identity. The Ministry of Agriculture veterinary investigation laboratories have available a slide agglutination test that can be used for this purpose. Further confirmatory evidence is gained by observation of the gross lesions of meningitis seen at post-mortem examination, i.e. oedema and congestion of the meningeal vasculature. See also Tables 8.1 and 8.2.

There may, in addition, be signs of arthritis, or serositis affecting the peritoneal cavity. The organism is difficult to grow once antibiotic treatment has commenced, but will normally grow on either horse or sheep's blood agar to produce small mucoid colonies surrounded by a narrow zone of haemolysis.

AETIOLOGY

Although the disease is present in a proportion of pig farms all over the UK there are many units that have remained free from the condition. The infection appears to enter the farm via infected carrier animals and to spread from them to the remainder of the herd (Table 8.3). Certain producers selling breeding stock are known to be infected and the herds that they supply inevitably contract the condition.

Herds without the disease should take great care to ensure that all stock purchased are derived from herds that are also known to be free of the disease. Affected animals are believed to carry the infection in the tonsils and transmission to the other pigs may well occur by the respiratory route.

Transmission experiments have shown that intravenous inoculation of *S. suis* type 2 will always cause infection whereas intranasal or pharyngeal transmission is somewhat less effective in passing on the disease. It may be supposed that a carrier sow infects its offspring shortly after birth. They in turn infect their pen mates when litters are grouped together at weaning. It has been shown that the organism can be recovered from 15 % of the tonsils of bacon pigs at the time of slaughter.

Humans can be infected with the disease and cases have been reported both in veterinary surgeons and in workers in slaughterhouses. The bacteria can survive in the nasal tract of man, and it is believed that they can, on occasions, be carried between farms by this route. Veterinary surgeons have generally agreed that although they move from infected to non-infected farms it is rare for a herd to develop the disease unless there is definite evidence of infected pigs being introduced to the farm.

Table 8.1 Typical signs and differential diagnosis of *S. suis* infections in pigs

	S. suis type 2	*S. suis* type 1	Aujeszky's disease	Bowel oedema	Salt poisoning	Arsenic toxicity
Age	1–16 weeks	2–6 weeks	0–12 weeks	3–12 weeks	All ages after weaning	All ages
Morbidity (%)	5–10	0–5	50–100	0–10	0–70	0–70
Mortality (%)	0–5	0–1	50–100	0–5	0–10	0–5
Nervous signs	+ + +	+	+ + +	+ +	+ + +	+ + +
Enteric signs	−	−	+	+ +	−	−
Respiratory signs	+	−	+	+	−	−

− Absent.
+ Mild.
+ + Moderate.
+ + + Severe.

Table 8.2 Causes of nervous signs in young pigs

Viral diseases
  Swine fever
  African swine fever
  Talfan disease

Bacterial diseases
  Escherichia coli meningitis
  Haemophilus species meningitis
  Salmonella species meningitis
  Tetanus
  Abscess formation in the spinal cord

Nutritional factors
  Malnutrition
  Water deprivation
  Vitamin A deficiency
  Nitrate and nitrite poisoning
  Pantothenic acid deficiency
  Nicotinic acid deficiency

Spinal damage

Table 8.3 Infections recorded in one veterinary practice 1979–1983

Farms under survey	104
Farms with S. *suis* type 2 present	28 (27 %)
Farms that contracted S. *suis* type 2 without purchasing infected pigs	2 (2 %)
Suspected cause	
Manager works on infected farm	1 (1 %)
Unknown	1 (1 %)

TREATMENT AND CONTROL

Following infection, a septicaemia develops; this lasts for 10–24 days. Not all pigs with septicaemia subsequently develop meningitis.

The treatment of meningitis poses many problems for the veterinary surgeon and it is a disease where the maxim "prevention is better than cure" certainly applies. The condition can be kept out of a herd free from it by judicious purchase of stock, which is a course of action to be strongly recommended.

Once the infection has entered a herd, a series of control measures should be applied to minimize its effects. It should be remembered, however, that as the disease will only occur sporadically, many actions will produce an apparently favourable response.

CONTROL MEASURES

These can be summarized as follows:

Maintain a high average age in the breeding animals for maximum immunity. Expand herd size gradually.
Reduce stress to the minimum.
Avoid overcrowding and keep animals in small groups.
Avoid extremes of temperature, dietary upsets and over- or underventilation.
Maintain a clean environment; do not allow dust to build up.
Remove clinical cases to a separate recovery area.

By maintaining a high overall age, it is possible to maximize the level of immunity in the sows; by introducing gilts in gradually, the sudden presence of many non-immunized and susceptible animals is avoided.

AIR SPACE AND VENTILATION

It would seem that the total weight of pigs in a given air space is a critical factor in determining the onset of clinical symptoms. If 100 20 kg pigs weigh 2000 kg, 14 days later the same pigs may each weigh 30 kg, a total of 3000 kg. If left in a constant air space, the ratio of weight to air volume will have increased by 50 %, which could be sufficient to trigger disease.

The volume of the house is not the only factor involved in this balance. Some piggeries are open fronted, some are mechanically ventilated. Ventilation rates vary greatly from winter to summer, with the winter level often only 10 % of the summer rate. With such variation, cross infection and

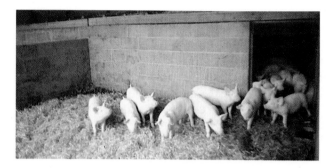

Fig. 8.1
Weaners bedded on
straw. Good
ventilation is
important for disease
control.

disease is always more likely at the lower level of ventilation.

The same events can occur in a kennel and yard system when, following a period of cold weather, the pigs may spend more time in the relatively unventilated and confined space of the kennel. In this context the build up of ammonia can often irritate the respiratory tract and trigger the appearance of clinical cases (Fig. 8.1).

Streptococci are relatively resistant to destruction and can survive in a room for periods of 1–2 months. Large areas of dust and dirt are likely to harbour the bacteria and initiate infection, so these should be cleared up (Fig. 8.2). Affected pigs are also likely to be exhaling the bacteria and are a source of infection to their pen mates so they are best removed to a separate area of the farm.

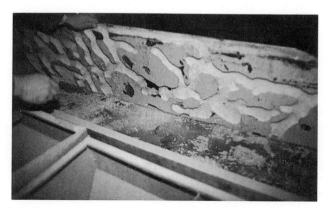

Fig. 8.2
Damage to insulation
and debris found
after a rat infestation.
Clean housing should
always be
maintained.

THERAPEUTIC MEASURES

Treatment and medication techniques for streptococcal meningitis are straightforward. The organism is usually sensitive to the penicillins and other antibiotics effective against Gram-positive organisms. As resistant *S. suis* type 2 have occasionally been reported, it is advisable to ensure that the organism is isolated and subjected to *in vitro* sensitivity tests if the response to treatment is not as expected.

Nursing

Clinical cases should be nursed with a great deal of care:

Remove them to a warm, dry, comfortable room, where self-mutilation is less likely to occur.
Administer parenteral antibiotics.
Ensure adequate fluid intakes. This is best achieved by intubation of the rectum and infusing an electrolyte solution (Blackburn, 1983).

With good nursing and early treatment, recovery rates are extremely high, but prompt treatment is essential (Table 8.4).

Table 8.4 Regimes used for the attempted control of *S. suis* type 2 infection

---

In-feed antibiotics to affected herds:
  Chlortetracycline
  Ampicillin
  Procaine penicillin (unstable)
  Potassium penicillin (unstable)

In-water antibiotics to affected herds

Parenteral injection of affected pigs

Nursing of affected pigs

Strategic oral or parenteral antibiotic medication timed to coincide with the likely occurrence of disease

Cleaning and disinfection of premises between batches of pigs

Antibiotic medication of batches of pigs after their move into cleaned premises as a preventive routine

Parenteral antibiotic treatment of sows before farrowing

Many veterinarians attempt to prevent and to treat the condition by in-feed medication with penicillin (220–400 g/t) or other antibiotics. In the author's experience the success of this technique is doubtful, especially as many of the penicillins deteriorate rapidly when placed in food or water supplies and then fail to produce adequate blood levels in the medicated pigs. There are no in-feed penicillins licensed for use in the UK and, although widely used, their efficacy is not proven.

When medication appears to work, its withdrawal may often be accompanied by the reappearance of clinical disease. Clinical disease can also occur during the period of medication.

Oral medication has been used in an attempt to produce populations free from the disease, but on most occasions, such efforts have been unsuccessful.

Carrier animals can be detected in populations being given in-feed penicillin. Parenteral administration of penicillin has been tried on many farms. On some, sows have been injected at the time of farrowing, and whole herds or groups within herds have been treated on others.

In humans, vaccination has been successful against forms of streptococcal meningitis. In pigs, despite substantial efforts, success has been limited, although work still continues in this area. It has been hampered by the relatively low financial importance of the disease.

A 100-sow herd producing 2000 pigs for sale each year would be expected to have a meningitis prevalence of no more than 2 % (40 pigs) of which 50 % would recover. This represents a financial cost (1983) of £550, a sum that is not likely to be sufficient to warrant any excessive expenditure on prevention or treatment.

On some occasions, the disease may become persistent, with a higher rate of infection. This usually coincides with poor environmental hygiene and a high level of concurrent disease.

CONCLUSION

S. *suis* type 2 infections have become established in many UK pig herds in the past 10 years. Although not usually of major financial importance, the disease has a demoralizing effect on staff, as well as affecting a significant proportion of pigs.

Control by vaccination or medication has not been outstand-ingly successful, but the adoption of good management and hygiene techniques, coupled with skilled nursing of affected pigs, has given good results. Farms that have removed the pigs, cleaned their premises and restocked 6 weeks later have been reported as remaining free from the disease.

REFERENCES

Blackburn, P. W. (1983). *Veterinary Record* **112,** 83.
De Moor, X. (1963). *Anatomie van Geeuwenock* **29,** 272.
Windsor, A. & Elliott, Y. (1975). *Journal of Hygiene Cambridge,* **75,** 69.

CHAPTER 9

Diagnosis of *Streptococcus suis* Infection in Pigs

FELICITY CLIFTON-HADLEY AND TOM ALEXANDER

INTRODUCTION

Streptococcus suis is subdivided into serotypes. Thirty have been recognized worldwide, but only types 1, 2 and a mixed type 1/2 are commonly identified in the UK. Of these, disease caused by type 2 is the most often diagnosed and the most damaging economically. Diseases due to types 1 and 1/2 are of minor importance. In other countries, different serotypes prevail. For example, in Denmark, type 7 is most frequently associated with disease. This article will deal mainly with the diagnosis of type 2 infection and only make brief mention of the others, but their diagnosis would follow similar lines.

CLINICAL PICTURE

A tentative diagnosis may be possible from the herd history and the typical clinical syndrome.

Disease due to *S. suis* type 1 tends to be confined to sucking pigs although it has been reported in weaned pigs up to 8 weeks of age. Disease due to other serotypes occurs in various ages of growing pigs. In contrast, the highest incidence of disease due to *S. suis* type 2 is in weaners of 5–10-weeks-old, particularly where they are housed intensively in large groups. In some herds, there may be a second peak in older growing pigs. The incidence varies between and within herds but rarely exceeds 5 %. Clinical cases are associated with stress factors such as mixing and moving, overcrowding, build-up of fumes from slurry and poor ventilation.

Streptococcus suis type 2 is the most common cause of meningitis in pigs in the UK. It also causes arthritis, septicaemia, polyserositis and endocarditis. In other parts of Europe and North America it is frequently associated with bronchopneumonia.

The most striking clinical sign is acute meningitis, which progresses rapidly to death unless treatment is given promptly. Pigs may be found dead with no premonitory signs. In less acute cases of meningitis, the first sign is a rise in rectal temperature to as high as 42.5°C (108°F) followed by inappetence, depression, reddening of the skin, adoption of unusual postures and incoordination. Within hours more obvious nervous signs develop including inability to stand, paddling, opisthotonus, convulsions and nystagmus. Fever, lameness, mild inappetence and depression may occur in the absence of meningitis and may go unrecognized.

POST-MORTEM FINDINGS

Although human cases are rare, it should be remembered when carrying out a post-mortem examination that *S. suis* type 2 can cause disease in people. Types 4 and 14 have also been recorded in people. Commonsense precautions should therefore be taken.

The lesions observed post mortem vary in severity and extent. Gross lesions may be minimal or absent even in pigs which had been lame and meningitic (Fig. 9.1). Typical gross findings, when present, include reddening of the skin, enlargement and congestion of lymph nodes, congestion of parenchymatous organs and a fibrinous polyserositis. In affected joints there may be thickening and reddening of the synovial membranes and excess clear, cloudy or purulent synovial fluid. Articular surfaces are not affected. In the central

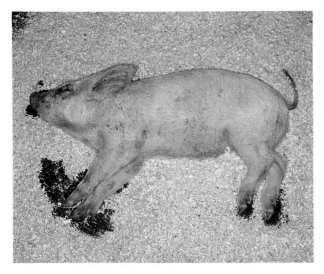

Fig. 9.1
Clinical case.

nervous system there may be thickening and congestion of the meninges (Fig. 9.2), congestion and oedema of the brain and excess purulent cerebrospinal fluid.

Where *S. suis* type 2 is associated with bronchopneumonia,

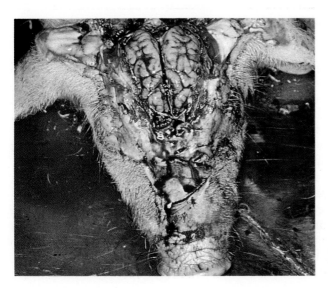

Fig. 9.2
Congested brain and meninges.

lesions are variable depending upon the other respiratory pathogens present and include lobular consolidation, interlobular emphysema, fibropurulent pleuritis, and mediastinal lymphadenopathy.

Valvular endocarditis may sometimes be caused by type 2. It is also associated with serotypes 1, 1/2, 7 or 8.

HISTOPATHOLOGICAL FINDINGS

Affected joints show changes of a proliferative fibrinous or fibrinopurulent synovitis with infiltration of neutrophils and mononuclear cells. In the central nervous system, changes are typical of an acute bacterial leptomeningitis with associated choroiditis and are characterized by a marked diffuse infiltration of neutrophils. In affected lungs there is usually a fibrinous or suppurative bronchopneumonia with occasionally perivascular, peribronchial and peribronchiolar accumulations of lymphocytes; interstitial pneumonia with giant cells in alveoli; bronchitis, bronchiolitis alveolar haemorrhage and necrosis.

BACTERIAL SMEARS

Smears are frequently omitted in routine diagnostic procedures but may be valuable in confirming the presence of streptococci, particularly if culturing fails (as may occur in a treated pig) and in providing a rapid interim diagnosis. On the other hand, a negative smear does not necessarily mean that the disease was not caused by *S. suis*. Smears are usually prepared from joints, meninges, brain and cerebrospinal fluid and examined for the presence of oval Gram-positive diplococci and short chains. (Aberrant pleomorphic forms are also occasionally seen.) Bacterial cells may be few while inflammatory cells are often abundant (Fig. 9.3). A preliminary identification of *S. suis* type 2 may be made by using direct or indirect fluorescent antibody test on smears from lesions (Fig. 9.4). As non-specific cross-reactions occur with other bacteria, fluorescent antibody tests are not conclusive and are unsuitable for use on mixed populations of bacteria (e.g. tonsil smears).

BACTERIOLOGICAL SAMPLING

Conclusive diagnosis depends upon the isolation of the organism in culture and its specific identification by serological tests. Samples are usually taken post mortem from the cerebrospinal fluid, brain, synovial fluid and heart blood but may also be taken from peritoneal, pleural and pericardial fluids and internal organs. Aseptic precautions should be used as contaminated samples may mask the presence of low numbers of *S. suis* organisms. Samples are grown overnight aerobically at 37°C on blood agar plates (Fig. 9.5). *S. suis* organisms grow as mucoid colonies with variable haemolytic patterns. Many, but not all, produce narrow zones of complete haemolysis on horse blood agar and partial haemolysis on calf or sheep blood agar. Growth and haemolysis are enhanced under anaerobic conditions. Colonies for identification are subcultured into Todd–Hewitt broth or similar enriched media. Single colonies often fail to grow when subcultured directly into broth and

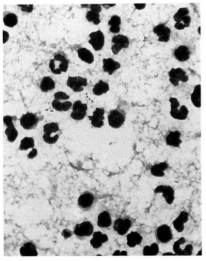

Fig. 9.3
Gram-stained smear of joint fluid showing few bacteria but many inflammatory cells.

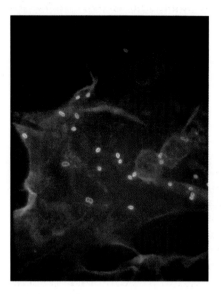

Fig. 9.4
Positive fluorescent-antibody test of cerebrospinal
fluid.

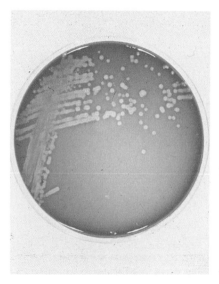

Fig. 9.5
Overnight aerobic culture on horse blood agar.

should first be subcultured onto blood agar plates to increase the inoculum.

SEROLOGICAL IDENTIFICATION

S. suis organisms belong to Lancefield's group D. The group D antigen is an intracellular lipid-bound teichoic acid which is difficult to extract and its demonstration is not normally undertaken for routine diagnosis. Diagnosis depends upon the demonstration of the type-specific polysaccharide capsular antigen (Fig. 9.6). Tests routinely used for this in the UK are the capsular reaction test, the precipitin test and the slide agglutination test (Fig. 9.7). In some other countries the coagglutination test is favoured and it is now starting to be tried in the UK. The advantages claimed for the coagglutination test, using latex beads or staphylococci, over the agglutination test are that it is more sensitive and more economical on sera. However, the precipitin test and capsular reaction test are the most accurate. The other two tests are slightly less reliable since cross reactions occur.

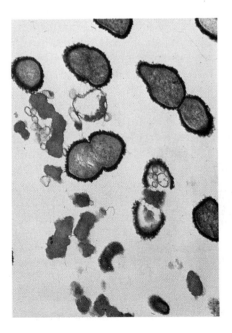

Fig. 9.6
Electromicrographs of *S. suis* type 2 showing the dark staining polysaccharide capsule.

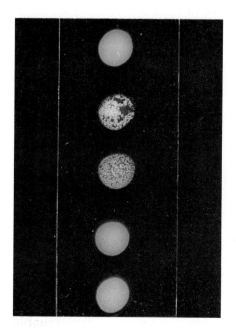

Fig. 9.7
Slide agglutination tests. From the top, the
second and middle samples are positive. The
rest are negative.

ANTISERA

Commercially available "group R" (i.e. type 2) diagnostic
antiserum is available but its continued supply is uncertain.
Hyperimmune antisera producing strong easily-read reactions
are readily prepared in rabbits. Doses (1 ml) of a formalin-
killed overnight Todd–Hewitt broth growth of *S. suis* washed
and resuspended in 0.85 % saline are injected intravenously
daily for 5 days. Courses are given in alternate weeks,
increasing the concentration of the injected suspension to four
times that of the original, until sera from test bleeds, when
examined in slide agglutination and precipitin tests with a
variety of streptococci, produce satisfactory positive and
negative reactions. Rabbits will provide high titre antiserum
for several years if booster injections are given as required.

CAPSULAR REACTION TEST

A 5–6 h culture of the suspected organism in serum (5 %)
broth is prepared to provide maximum capsule. Two loopfuls

are placed on a slide. A loopful of type specific antiserum is mixed into one and a loopful of control antiserum is mixed into the other. They are then compared under coverslips by ×1000 direct phase-contrast oil-immersion microscopy. If positive, the streptococci appear twice as big as those of the control.

PRECIPITIN TEST

Acid extracts are prepared by heating the centrifuged deposit (3500 g for 15 min) from 20 ml of overnight broth growth in 1 ml of 0.02N hydrochloric acid in 0.85 % sodium chloride solution (0.2 % hydrochloric acid, pH 2.5) at 100°C for 3 min. The type antigens of types 2, 7 and 8 are destroyed by heating in stronger acid (0.2N hydrochloric acid). The extracts are cooled and neutralized with normal sodium hydroxide after adding 1 drop of phenol red indicator (0.02 %, BDH, Poole, Dorset). Equal quantities of antiserum and centrifuged, neutralized extract are drawn up and sealed in capillary tubes and examined after a few minutes for precipitation. Negative reactions are checked after 30 min.

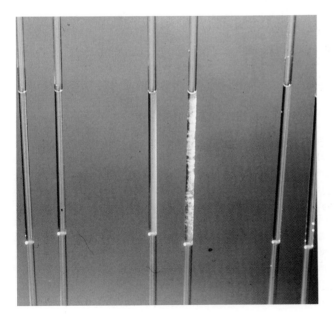

Fig. 9.8
Precipitin tests in capillary tubes. The two central tubes are positive.

SLIDE AGGLUTINATION TEST

Using a platinum wire loop, different antisera are added to drops of a smooth, heavy suspension of the centrifuged streptococci from an overnight broth culture on a glass microscope slide and mixed by rocking the slide gently on its longitudinal axis. A positive reaction is indicated in a few seconds by visible clumps forming in a clear liquid. A negative reaction leaves the suspension unchanged. Uneven suspensions of streptococci cannot be used in this test. Several sera are used in order to identify any non-specific positive reactions.

BIOCHEMICAL TESTS

Some diagnostic laboratories use commercially available galleries of biochemical tests instead of serological tests to identify *S. suis* type 2, but biochemical tests are not type-specific. A limited number of biochemical tests have been proposed for the presumptive diagnosis of the species *Streptococcus suis*. These include no growth in 6.5 % sodium chloride, a negative Voges–Proskauer test, and production of acid in trehalose and salicin broths, although some isolates are negative for one or other of these last two tests.

SCREENING HERDS FOR *S. SUIS* TYPE 2

Because of the seriousness of *S. suis* type 2 in some herds and because it can exist subclinically in others without the typical clinical syndrome being apparent, it would be useful in relation to the sale of breeding stock or weaners if there were a simple practical method for screening herds. Blood sampling and tonsil swabbing (or scraping) have both been considered.

None of the numerous blood tests that have been tried have proved specific. They have all cross-reacted with other bacteria and given false positive results in pigs which are not infected with *S. suis* type 2. Perhaps in the future, the use of monoclonal antibodies against specific epitopes may prove more specific.

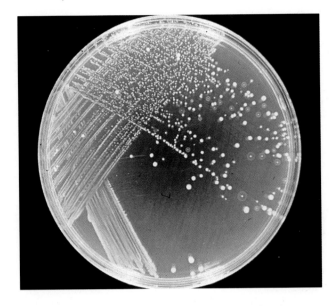

Fig. 9.9
Overnight aerobic culture on semi-selective serum agar from a tonsil swab. *S.suis* type 2 colonies are surrounded with faint but distinct haloes of precipitation.

Screening herds for tonsil carriers has been more promising. The organism has been detected in the tonsils of healthy pigs from apparently uninfected herds using a semi-selective serum agar medium. This medium contains high titre anti-*S. suis* type 2 antiserum and produces distinct haloes of precipitation around *S. suis* type 2 colonies (Fig. 9.9). However, some of these isolates have proved to be non-pathogenic or of low pathogenicity for pigs. Until recently virulence could only be determined by inoculating pigs experimentally. This is not only expensive and laborious but also unacceptable on welfare grounds for routine use. Dutch workers, (Vecht *et al.*, 1990) have reported a laboratory test for a muramidase-released-protein on *S. suis* type 2 the presence of which seems to be associated with virulence. This should make tonsil swabbing more useful but one still cannot forecast whether an isolate of low pathogenicity might mutate to become more virulent. It is therefore problematical to assess the significance of a positive tonsil culture from a herd showing no typical clinical signs. The usual method of assessment is to rely on the presence or absence of naturally occurring typical clinical cases from which *S. suis* type 2 can be isolated and identified.

REFERENCES AND FURTHER READING

Clifton-Hadley, F. A., Alexander, T. J. L. & Enright, M. R. (1985). *Pig Veterinary Society Proceedings* **14**, 27–34.
Higgins, R. & Gottschalk, N. (1990). *International Pig Veterinary Society Proceedings* (Lausanne), 169.
Vecht, V., Wisselink, H. J., Van Dijk, J. E. & Smith, H. E. (1990). *International Pig Veterinary Society Proceedings* (Lausanne), 173.

CHAPTER 10

Locomotor Disorders of the Pig

G. A. H. WELLS

INTRODUCTION

A specific diagnostic challenge is commonly posed by pigs with disorders which present as lameness or other locomotor signs.

Clinical entities and their differential diagnoses are listed in Tables 10.1–10.4 according to age incidence and location of lesions. Those conditions which occur relatively frequently in the United Kingdom are shown in bold type.

CLINICAL HISTORY, GENERAL INSPECTION AND PHYSICAL EXAMINATION

As in all competent investigations of disease the clinician must examine the history objectively and in detail. Affected pigs are identified and inspected in relationship to their specific husbandry system. The time course of the illness is noted. Simple observation of the pigs in their usual environment should define the basic problem as one of locomotor disability. A more detailed cháracterization and interpretation of clinical signs can then proceed.

Table 10.1 Clinical locomotor disorders of the pig according to location of lesions at 0–7 days of age

Nervous	Bones	Foot/tendons
Enterovirus encephalomyelitis (Teschen/Talfan)	Maternal vitamin A deficiency (osteodysgenesis)	Foot-and-mouth disease
Aujeszky's disease	Thickleg (hyperostosis/diaphyseal dysplasia)	Swine vesicular disease
Swine fever (Hog cholera)		Dermatosis vegetans
African swine fever		**Trauma/necrosis**
Haemagglutinating encephalomyelitis		
Bacterial meningoencephalitis	**Joints**	**Muscle**
Streptococcus suis I	**Neonatal polyarthritis**	Iron-induced myodegeneration (vitamin E deficiency)
Streptococcus suis II	Streptococcus species	**Splayleg**
Escherichia coli	Staphylococcus species	
Salmonella species	Escherichia coli	
Listeria monocytogenes	Haemophilus species	
Haemophilus parasuis		
Otoencephalitis		
Streptococcus species		
Pasteurella multocida		
Corynebacterium pyogenes		
Tetanus		
Sciatic nerve trauma/neuritis		
Congenital tremor (Cerebellar dysgenesis/cerebrospinal hypomyelinogenesis)		
Hypoxia		
Hypoglycaemia		
Hypothermia		

Disorders shown in bold type are common in occurrence.

Table 10.2 Clinical locomotor disorders of the pig according to location of lesions at 7 days of age to weaning

	Nervous	Joints	Bones	Foot/tendons
	Otoencephalitis *Streptococcus* species *Pasteurella multocida* *Corynebacterium pyogenes* Tetanus Copper deficiency myelopathy (>2 w) Vitamin A deficiency (<2 w)	**Neonatal polyarthritis** (1–2 w) *Streptococcus* species *Staphylococcus* species *Escherichia coli* *Haemophilus* species *Mycoplasma* polyserositis *Mycoplasma hyorhinus* (3–10 w) Glasser's disease *Haemophilus parasius* Actinobacillosis (1–6 w)	Rickets (2–10 w) Maternal vitamin A deficiency (osteodysgenesis) 'Kyphosis' (idiopathic)	Foot-and-mouth disease Swine vesicular disease Dermatosis vegetans (<6 w) Ergotism **Trauma/necrosis**
	Enterovirus encephalomyelitis (Teschen/Talfan) Aujeszky's disease Swine fever (Hog cholera) African swine fever Haemagglutinating encephalomyelitis (<2 w) Porcine cyto-megalovirus encephalitis **Bacterial meningoencephalitis** *Streptococcus suis* I (10–14d) *Streptococcus suis* II *Escherichia coli* (<14 d) *Salmonella* species *Listeria monocytogenes* *Haemophilus parasuis* (2 w–4 m)			Muscle Iron-induced myodegeneration (vitamin E deficiency) Nutritional muscular dystrophy (vitamin E/selenium deficiency) (>2 w) Pietrain creeper syndrome (3–8 w)

d, Days; w, Weeks; m, Months; Age range of incidence.
Disorders shown in bold type are common in occurrence.

Table 10.3 Clinical locomotor disorders of the pig according to location of lesions in weaned piglets

Nervous	Joints	Muscle	Foot/tendons
Epidural abscess	**Mycoplasma polyserositis**	Back muscle necrosis	Foot-and-mouth disease
Water deprivation/salt intoxication	*Mycoplasma hyorhinus* (3–10 w)	Asymmetric hindquarter, syndrome	Swine vesicular disease
Organoarsenical intoxication	**Mycoplasma arthritis**	**Porcine stress syndrome**	? Biotin deficiency (>3 m)
Organophosphorus intoxication	*Mycoplasma hyosynoviae* (8–24 w)	Nutritional muscular dystrophy (white muscle disease) (>2 w)	**Trauma/sepsis** (foot rot)
Focal symmetrical poliomyelomalacia (selenium intoxication) (6–10 w)	**Erysipelas arthritis** *Erysipelothrix rhusiopathiae* (12–24 w)	Monensin/tiamulin intoxication (myodegeneration)	**Bursitis**
Alkyl mercury intoxication	**Streptococcal arthritis**	Pietrain creeper syndrome (3–8 w)	Bones
Furazolidone intoxication	Glasser's disease *Haemophilus parasuis* (5–8 w)		Rickets (2–10 w)
Enterovirus encephalomyelitis (Teschen/Talfan) (<12 w)			**Osteochondrosis/ osteoarthrosis** (>4 m)
Aujeszky's disease (<2 m)			
Swine fever (Hog choleral)			
African swine fever			
Swine vesicular disease encephalitis			
Bacterial meningoencephalitis *Streptococcus suis II* (3–12 w)			

Listeria monocytogenes	Vitamin A deficiency	Actinobacillosis	"Kyphosis" (idiopathic)
Salmonella species	Pantothenic acid deficiency	Discospondylitis	Fractures – trauma; (electrocution)
Haemophilus parasuis (2 w–4 m)	Copper deficiency myelopathy (>2 w)	*Erysipelothrix insidiosa*	Osteomyelitis
Otoencephalitis	Cerebrospinal lipodystrophy (3 m)	Spondylosis	
Streptococcus species	Fibrocartilaginous embolism of spinal cord	**Osteoarthrosis**	
Pasteurella multocida	Hypoxia (cardiac insufficiency) (nitrate/nitrite intoxication)		
Corynebacterium pyogenes	Heat stroke		
Tetanus			
Oedema disease/CSA (4–12 w)			

w, Weeks; m, Months; Age range of incidence.
Disorders shown in bold type are common in occurrence.

Table 10.4 Clinical locomotor disorders of the pig according to location of lesions in adult pigs

Nervous	Bones	Muscle	Foot/tendons
Enterovirus encephalomyelitis (Teschen)	**Osteochondrosis/ osteoarthrosis**	Back muscle necrosis	Foot-and-mouth disease
Swine fever (Hog cholera)	**Epiphyseolysis/ apophyseolysis** (5 m–3 y)	Asymmetric hindquarter syndrome	Swine vesicular disease
African swine fever	Osteomalacia/ osteoporosis (fractures in lactating/weaned sows)	**Porcine stress syndrome**	? Biotin deficiency
Swine vesicular disease encephalitis		Haematoma (haemorrhagic diatheis)	**Trauma/sepsis** (foot rot)
Bacterial meningencephalitis	"Kyphosis" (idiopathic)	Warfarin/coumarol	**Overgrown hooves**
Streptococcus suis II	Fractures – trauma; (electrocution)	? mycotoxins	Laminitis (boars) and sows recently farrowed)
Haemophilus parasuis	Osteomyelitis		**Bursitis**
Heat stroke			
Otoencephalitis	Joints		
Streptococcus species	Mycoplasma arthritis		
Pasteurella multocida	*Mycoplasma hyosynoviae*		
Corynebacterium pyogenes	**Erysipelas arthritis**		
Epidural abscess	*Erysipelothrix rhusiopathiae*		
Brain abscess	Streptococcal arthritis		
Water deprivation/ salt intoxication	Glasser's disease - *Haemophilus parasuis*		
Organoarsenical intoxication	Discospondylitis		
Alkyl mercury intoxication	*Erysipelothrix rhusiopathiae*		
Organophosphorus intoxication	Spondylosis		
Adult Landrace trembles (>3 m)	**Osteoarthrosis**		
	Tarsitis		

m, Months; y, Years; Age range of incidence.

Affected animals should be singled out and observed in good light moving about on a clean, dry and level surface. Pigs are not amenable to handling and so detailed physical examination should be deferred until the inspection and assessment of behaviour has been completed with minimal interference.

The next stage is to confine the pig so as to carry out superficial palpation of limbs, joints and muscles. With placid adults this may be achieved by simply coaxing them into a corner. If possible, manipulation of the limbs should then also be performed on the free-standing animal.

Restraint is finally necessary to examine the feet, systematically starting with the sole of the foot and working proximally, and to complete detailed palpation and manipulation of the limbs.

LAMENESS

Lameness can be defined as impaired movement or deviation from normal gait. More frequently in the veterinary context lameness refers to abnormal gait caused by painful lesions of the limbs or back; also to mechanical limb defects. Neurological deficits which none the less produce lameness are usually defined separately.

Lameness caused by pain should be readily recognized during a general clinical examination but certain musculoskeletal disorders and indeed some systemic diseases may resemble primary nervous conditions in their clinical presentation.

A basic neurological examination is therefore often required and in practice can be incorporated into the general clinical examination. Clinical neurology relates abnormal nervous function to anatomic site of damage thus seeking to localize the lesion but does not contribute greatly towards an aetiological diagnosis.

NEUROLOGICAL EXAMINATION AND CLINICAL INTERPRETATIONS

In pigs the art of clinical neurology is not well developed. Nevertheless, the clinician should seek to extend basic observations whenever the occasion presents in order to acquire an essential appreciation of the normal response. A checklist of examination procedures (see further reading) is an invaluable aid. Clearly there are limitations in dealing with large pigs.

When considering locomotor aspects of central nervous and neuromuscular diseases it is a useful concept to divide clinical neurological signs into so-called "head" signs, those indicative of intracranial or brain disease and those suggesting extracranial nervous disease. "Head" signs include changes in mental state, seizures or convulsions, abnormal head posture, incoordination of head movement and cranial nerve deficits.

The absence of "head" signs in neurological disease suggests that the lesion is caudal to the foramen magnum, in the spinal cord, peripheral nerves or skeletal muscles. Frequently some "head" signs will accompany presenting abnormalities of posture and gait. This should immediately arouse suspicion of multifocal, diffuse or systematic distribution of nervous system lesions.

"HEAD" SIGNS AND LOCOMOTION

Alterations of mental state such as depression, disorientation, coma or hyperexcitability may accompany locomotor signs. Depression and disorientation are features of the non-suppurative viral encephalitides, Aujeszky's disease and haemagglutinating encephalomyelitis. A "euphoric" state is reported to occur in pigs poisoned with arsanilic acid. Hyperexcitability is the initial feature of toxicity from another organoarsenical feed additive, 3-nitro. Later in the course of that poisoning, continued overdosage produces cases with paraparesis and paraplegia. Hyperexcitability is also seen in enterovirus encephalomyelitis.

A progression through disorientation to seizures or fits is seen in many inflammatory conditions of the brain and its coverings. Most common of these is bacterial meningitis. Seizures are characterized by marked diffuse increase in muscle tone, falling into lateral recumbency and rhythmic clonic convulsions simulating running or pedalling movements of the limbs. Depression or even coma may follow a seizure.

Opisthotonus (dorsiflexion of the neck) with extension of the limbs is also seen with meningitis.

There are several metabolic and other systemic disorders of pigs which, as in other species, have secondary effects upon the central nervous system including serious locomotor deficits. Their primary pathophysiology is not within the locomotor apparatus. Nervous signs of generalized metabolic derangement are often mediated via the blood–brain barrier. The effects on the central nervous system are therefore often intermittent, always generalized and produce a wide spectrum of inconstant neurological signs, mostly "head" signs. These include confusion, coma, syncope, collapse, seizures, tremors, vision disturbances, quadriparesis, paraparesis and episodic weakness.

Hypoglycaemia, though not a specific disease, is frequently the main metabolic manifestation of starvation in piglets during the first week of life. Confusion and ataxia progress to quadriparesis, sometimes seizures and to death in coma. In the ataxic stages piglets stand base wide and may rest their noses upon the floor apparently to gain further support. Hypoxia of the central nervous system can result from nitrate/nitrite poisoning, from airway obstructions associated with severe coughing and from cardiac insufficiency.

Cardiac insufficiency in turn can result from piglet anaemia, mulberry heart disease and bacterial endocarditis. Progressive apathy, coma and death from cardiac arrest occur with hyperkalaemia in cases of parenteral iron-induced myodegeneration of the vitamin E deficient piglet.

In the porcine stress syndrome acidosis plays a significant role in the clinical disease but clearly does not account for all the observed signs. The syndrome has been described as heralded by a rapid tremor of the tail but this is often not observed. Dyspnoea, reluctance to move, muscular weakness, collapse, tremors, muscular rigidity, cyanosis and death follow. Also in the earlier stages characteristic shifting areas of erythema and pallor are seen on the skin. Hyperthermia is an essential feature of porcine stress syndrome. Heat stroke occurs only in pigs exposed to high ambient temperatures. Signs resemble those in porcine stress syndrome but without muscular rigidity.

POSTURE

Postural abnormalities are present both in nervous diseases and in musculoskeletal and foot problems. While noting posture, the conformation of the pig can also be assessed. Asymmetric hindquarter syndrome presents without lameness but with very marked disproportion of the proximal musculature of the hindlimbs.

Similarly in an idiopathic spinal curvature provisionally termed "humped back and dipped shoulders syndrome" and seen at several different ages, pigs do not show locomotor deficits, only the obvious spinal curvature (Fig. 10.1). Probably of little economic importance in fattening pigs, this condition is clearly a serious potential problem when it occurs occasionally in gilts reared for replacement of breeding stock.

Kyphosis often associated with limb lameness is seen in spondylosis and discospondylitis. Arching of the back, a voluntary movement seemingly to minimize both skeletal and abdominal pain, is common in arthritis of limb joints. Curvature (pleurothotonus) of the body is seen in back muscle necrosis when the lesion is unilateral. The affected side forms the convexity of the curvature.

Abnormal carriage of the head is often a sign of cerebellar or vestibular disease. Involvement of the vestibular nerve, vestibular nucleus or flocculonodular lobe of the cerebellum should be suspected when a head tilt is present. Unilateral head tilt is usually present in otoencephalitis. Facial nerve paralysis occurs sometimes with this condition to give a

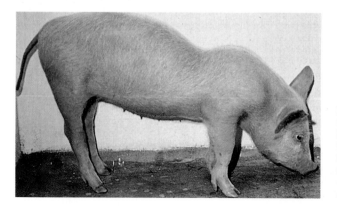

Fig. 10.1
Idiopathic lumbar kyphosis, thoracic lordosis ("humped back dipped shoulders syndrome") – an acquired spinal curvature.

drooping ear on the affected side. Leaning or falling to the affected side may also occur.

A wide-based stance is characteristic of cerebellar dysfunction. Pleurothotonus and a tendency to circle, without difficulty in standing, is seen with forebrain lesions.

Abnormalities of posture in recumbent animals may indicate paralysis or muscular weakness. Paraplegia in the pig causes a sitting posture (Fig. 10.2). If spasticity is present the limbs are extended forward.

Pain in a limb will produce abnormal limb positioning; often flexion or abduction to avoid weight bearing. Shifting of weight from one leg to another in the standing position is seen in polyarthritis. When there is pain involving all four feet as in aseptic laminitis of breeding adults, a posture is adopted with the back arched and the feet bunched together under the abdomen. Such animals are reluctant to move. A similar stance is typical of chronic erysipelas arthritis of the older pig (Fig. 10.3).

A wide variety of abnormalities of limb shape and angulation have been described in so-called leg weakness of rapidly growing young pigs. Clinical lameness in this disorder is considered to be related to the development of degenerative joint change (osteoarthrosis) though frequently the underlying change, osteochondrosis, is a disturbance of endochondral ossification. Limb conformation changes variably include hyperflexion of the carpus (in the standing posture) so that the centre of gravity is taken forwards forcing weight to be taken through the toe, adduction of the forelimbs below the carpus ("knock knee"), hyperextension of the phalanges, lateral angulation of the lower hindleg and curvature of the tarsus,

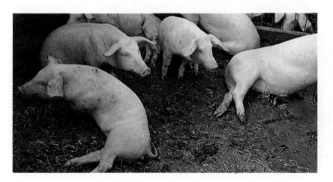

Fig. 10.2
Paraplegia in fattening pigs caused by organophosphorus neurotoxicity. Upper and lower motor neurones and long spinal proprioceptive tracts are all affected.

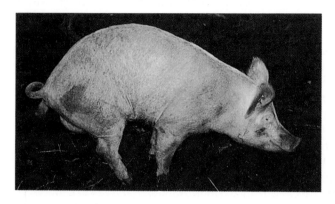

Fig. 10.3
Chronic erysipelas
arthritis in an 18-
month-old boar. Note
the arched back and
feet bunched
together.

or straightness of the hindlimb. Gait abnormalities also occur including crossing of the hindlegs and swaying of the hindquarters (Fig. 10.4).

MOVEMENT

Disordered movement in the context of locomotor diseases means alterations in gait, though tremors can also affect locomotion. Gait deficits are not usually associated with lesions rostral to the midbrain. In the absence of "head" signs further

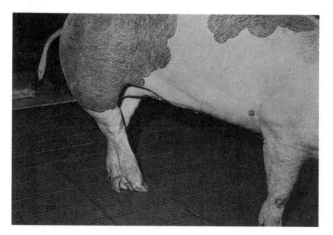

Fig. 10.4
Crossed hindlegs
associated with "leg
weakness" in a gilt.

localization can be achieved with reference to limb signs (Table 10.5).

Ataxia means incoordination of muscular action or gait. Signs include wide-based stance, swaying movements of the trunk, falling, rolling, dysmetria (imprecise excursion of movement), crossing of the limbs and exaggerated abduction of the limbs on turning. Ataxia is one of the most common clinical signs in porcine nervous diseases. Clearly it cannot be appreciated in the presence of paralysis.

The localization of changes causing ataxia can be differentiated clinically (Table 10.6). Some encephalitides, for example that of swine fever, present with ataxia, referable to hindbrain lesions. Sensory ataxia results from selective loss of proprioception.

Proprioception is the animal's ability to recognize the location of its limbs in relation to the rest of the body. Long tracts, relaying sensory information to the brain from the limbs, are to be found in the dorsal columns and in the lateral columns (spinocerebellar) of the spinal cord. Selective damage to these tracts is seen in organophosphorus neurotoxicity, 3-nitro intoxication and pantothenic acid deficiency (Fig. 10.5). More severe ataxia is seen with selective spinocerebellar tract damage than with dorsal column lesions. Dorsal column tracts, however, project to the cerebral cortex and are therefore responsible for conscious proprioception. Knuckling of the lower limbs (fetlocks) is the major sign of deficits in conscious proprioception.

Dysmetria may take the form of movements that are too long (hypermetria) or too short (hypometria). Hypermetria,

Table 10.5 Location of lesions from gait deficits without "head" signs

All limbs involved	Hindlimbs only involved
Focal – cervical spinal cord	Focal, multifocal or diffuse – thoracolumbar spinal cord
Diffuse or multifocal – spinal cord	
Diffuse – peripheral nerves	Bilateral – peripheral nerves (lumbosacral plexus projections)
Diffuse – neuromuscular junction	
Diffuse – skeletal muscle	Skeletal muscles

Table 10.6 Neurological differential localization of ataxia

Neurological sign	Sensory ataxia (afferent proprioceptive tracts)		Cerebellar ataxia (Motor)	Vestibular ataxia	
	Hindbrain (excluding vestibular)	Spinal cord		Central	Peripheral
Altered mental status	+	–	–	+	–
Head involvement (e.g. tilt or tremor)	+	–	++	+	+
Tremors	–	–	++	–	–
Nystagmus (involuntary rhythmic eye movements)	–	–	+	+	+
Postural reaction deficits					
on initiation	+	+	–	+	–
on follow-through	+	++	++	+	–
Symmetrical deficits	–	++	++	+	–
Hypermetric gait	+	++	+	±	–

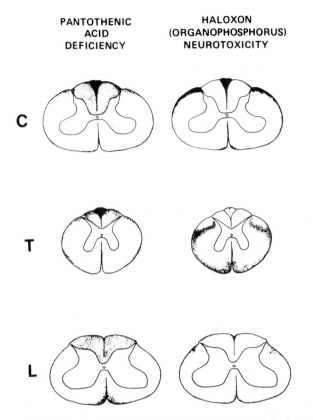

PANTOTHENIC
ACID
DEFICIENCY

HALOXON
(ORGANOPHOSPHORUS)
NEUROTOXICITY

Fig. 10.5 Diagrammatic distribution of spinal cord long fibre tract degeneration in organophosphorus neurotoxicity and panthothenic acid deficiency. Note dorsal column (conscious proprioception) lesions in both at the cervical level (C). Spinocerebellar tracts are also affected in organophosphorus neurotoxicity. T, thoracic level; L, lumbar level.

often called "goose-stepping" is a relatively common sign in the pig. It is the main presenting sign together with some swaying of the body in pantothenic acid deficiency, which is now relatively rare (Fig. 10.6). Hypermetria is also seen occasionally in Aujeszky's disease, in epidemic streptococcal meningitis with spinal cord involvement and in furazolidone poisoning. Ankylosis of the tarsus, seen sometimes as part of the osteochondrosis/osteoarthrosis complex will for mechanical reasons rather than proprioceptive deficits also produce a jerky stiff hindleg gait resembling "goose-stepping".

Assessment of gait should take account of length of stride. A dysmetric gait often includes a long stride, a prolonged

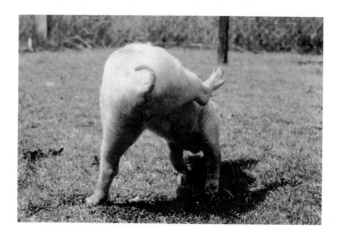

Fig. 10.6
Pantothenic acid
deficiency –
hypermetria (goose-
stepping).

supporting phase and is bilateral. In contrast painful musculoskeletal or foot lesions give a short stride, a reduced support
phase and are often unilateral.

Ataxia is usually absent in musculoskeletal diseases and in
diseases which affect the motor fibres of peripheral nerves
but frequently the presenting sign in the latter will be paresis
or paralysis.

Paralysis can be defined as loss of motor or sensory nerve
function. Paresis is partial paralysis. Muscular weakness
caused by a primary muscle lesion, as in the myodegeneration
resulting from an interaction between tiamulin and monensin
used therapeutically in conjunction, will present as apparent
quadriparesis and in practice may be indistinguishable from
true neurogenic paresis. In such cases when a neurogenic
component of the "paralysis" can be ruled out the term
muscular weakness is more appropriate than paralysis. Primary
muscle diseases are usually associated with postural or exer-
tional weakness of muscles, stiffness, muscle pain and changes
in size of muscles (atrophy or hypertrophy). For the clinical
assessment of spinal cord and peripheral nervous system
motor deficits it is conventional to consider two functional
units, the lower motor neurone and the upper motor neurone
(Table 10.7).

Located in the ventral horns of the spinal cord grey matter
and in the brain stem (cranial nerve motor nuclei) the lower
motor neurone is the effector neurone. Lower motor neurone

Table 10.7 Spinal cord and peripheral nervous system motor deficits

	Lower motor neurone (PNS)	Upper motor neurone (CNS)
Paresis/paralysis	Mild to severe	Mild to severe
Spinal reflexes	Decreased	Normal, altered or increased
Muscle atrophy	Severe (neurogenic) [2–3 weeks]	Mild (disuse) [? months]
Muscle tone	Decreased	Decreased, normal or hypertonic (spasticity)

nerve fibres extend as the peripheral nervous system to innervate skeletal muscle and are the final common pathway for both voluntary and reflex movement. The lower motor neurone together with its corresponding primary sensory neurone in the spinal dorsal root ganglia provides therefore a means of testing spinal reflexes.

In the pig the concept of a single upper motor neurone continuous from the cerebral motor cortex to the lower motor neurone is not valid, for although the pathway exists it is formed by a relay of many interneurones. Nevertheless to consider the upper motor neurone as a functional unit providing higher central nervous system control is still useful in the understanding of spinal cord and peripheral nerve disorders.

Differentiation and localization of upper and lower motor neurone damage clinically is simplistically based on the assumption that a single focal lesion interrupts the neuroaxis. In the pig such lesions include vertebral fracture, epidural abscess and fibrocartilaginous embolism of the spinal cord.

When diffuse or multifocal intracranial disease is present upper and lower motor neurone deficits may be obscured by "head" signs. Multifocal upper motor neurone lesions give signs indistinguishable from a single lesion at the most rostral point of damage. Concurrent upper and lower motor neurone lesions will display signs consistent with damage to only the lowest (most distal) lesion on the neuroaxis, i.e. the lower motorneurone lesion, since this is the final common pathway of limb innervation.

In enterovirus encephalomyelitis concurrent upper and lower motor neurone lesions occur but the presenting signs may be confined to paraplegia or quadriplegia without upper motor neurone signs. Quadriplegia with lower motor neurone features is also the main presenting sign in focal poliomyelomalacia associated with selenium intoxication.

Tremor

Tremor is a regular abnormal movement caused by involuntary changes in muscle tone. It is seen sometimes in diffuse brain diseases, in particular viral encephalitides, when the tremor can be violent, but is often accompanied by "head" signs.

Congenital diffuse myelin disorders produce generalized tremors in piglets at or near birth. While the piglet is active the trembling is constant but it subsides at rest. Severely affected piglets can tremble so violently that they are unable to suck. An idiopathic tremor, intermittent in form and associated also with movement, particularly enforced walking backwards, is seen in some adolescent Landrace pigs. This condition sometimes resolves spontaneously after a few months.

Generalized tremor is also present in neuromuscular weakness and this may be the explanation for tremor in a hereditary myopathy of the Pietrain breed; so-called Pietrain creeper syndrome.

A sustained or continuous tremor can be induced experimentally in ruminants and pigs by the administration of certain mycotoxins. Tremorgenic mycotoxins have been proposed as the cause of several so-called "stagger" ataxias which occur naturally in ruminants. Although no similar disorders have been reported in pigs, State veterinary service colleagues have described one disease outbreak in which gilts housed in a walled garden developed an episodic tremor and forelimb weakness (Fig. 10.7). Mouse bioassay tests of soil extracts demonstrated a neurotoxic principle. Complete recovery occurred within 48 h of moving the pigs to a concrete yard.

In tetanus there is generalized muscle contraction (spasm) brought about by the effects of tetanus toxin absorbed into the central and peripheral nervous systems. If muscle spasms are prolonged they are termed "tonic" and if rapid they are

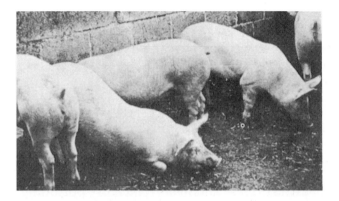

Fig. 10.7
Suspected
mycotoxicosis.
Episodic weakness
and collapse of
forelimbs associated
with intermittent
tremor in pigs kept in
an old walled
garden.

termed "clonic". In tetanus the spasms are largely tonic with intermittent clonus. There is hyperaesthesia and external stimuli exacerbate the signs. In pigs, signs progress over 1–2 days from a stiff gait to lateral recumbency with opisthotonos and extensor rigidity of all limbs. The ears are erect and there is elevation of the tail.

Muscle spasm also occurs in generalized seizures but the tonic phase is usually brief and it is clonic limb movements of running or pedalling that are characteristic.

POSTURAL REACTIONS

Standard testing methods are employed in small companion animal neurology to assess the competence of the sensory (conscious proprioception) and motor systems to perform smooth, coordinated complex movements. They do not give the clinician information on the localization of the lesion, are difficult to perform in pigs and in the absence of data for the species also difficult to interpret.

Proprioceptive positioning of the limbs is effected through touch (sensory) and muscle (motor) activity and can be tested by placing the dorsal aspect of the foot on the ground. Immediate replacement of the foot to the normal position should occur. A proprioceptive deficit is indicated by the foot remaining in the knuckled over position. This may have already been suspected from the observation of knuckling during natural movement. Sciatic and fibular nerve damage will also produce knuckling over of the foot and must be distinguished from long spinal tract proprioceptive deficits. In exclusively peripheral nerve lesions there is no ataxia.

Other postural reflex tests which can be usefully performed in the young pig include wheelbarrowing, swaying, extensor thrust and placing.

CRANIAL NERVE EXAMINATIONS

Vision defects affect locomotion. They occur in organoarsenical poisoning, in the focal encephalomalacia and cerebrospinal angiopathy of oedema disease and in alkyl mercury poisoning, also variably in enterovirus encephalomyelitis, bacterial meningitis and water deprivation encephalopathy. Assessment of vision deficits in the pig must be based mainly upon observations of behaviour. Failure to avoid unfamiliar objects, especially in poor light, is the main criterion.

Vestibular disease, both central and peripheral, is important in the differential causes of ataxia.

SPINAL REFLEXES

Spinal reflexes can be tested only to a limited extent in the pig. Tests provide assessment of the spinal reflex arcs and the lower motor neurones supplying the limbs and the influence of higher centre changes on the reflex arcs. The patellar myotatic or knee jerk reflex can be tested in the young pig. The pig is held in lateral recumbency and is allowed to relax before testing. The straight patellar ligament is tapped with a suitable size of neurological percussion hammer.

In older paralysed pigs the test can also be performed. A decreased or absent response indicates loss of lower motor neurone or sensory relay function of the reflex arc. An exaggerated reflex is caused by release of the reflex from higher (upper motor neurone) inhibitory influences. Because these pathways are inhibitory to extensor muscles and facilitatory to flexor muscles an exaggerated patellar reflex is often accompanied by extensor hypertonia or spasticity.

The flexor (pedal or withdrawal) reflex can be performed on the partly extended limbs by pinching the claws or the interdigital skin with the pig in lateral recumbency. Only the minimum force required to evoke a reaction need be applied. Flexion of the whole limb is considered a normal response. The reflex involves those spinal cord segments supplying the lower motor neurones of the main peripheral nerves of the limb under test. Lesions within the appropriate cord segments, spinal nerve roots or peripheral nerves will cause deficits.

PALPATION AND MANIPULATION

This part of the examination is of greatest importance in the localization of musculoskeletal disorders. Palpation will include evaluation of muscle tone, muscle size, determining atrophy or hypertrophy, and muscle consistency. In acute back muscle necrosis the longissimus dorsi muscle is swollen and firm, but in more chronic cases, atrophic and hard. Swellings are palpated. Heat can be detected in acute inflammatory lesions. In limb lameness the mobility and excursion of joint movement should be checked. Crepitus may be detected on manipulation of fractured long bones but is rarely elicited from vertebral fractures. Separation of the proximal femoral epiphysis (epiphyseolysis) or separation of the ischial tuberosity (apophyseolysis) may be palpable.

The examination of the foot should note particularly discolorations, heat or swelling, separations of sole or hoof wall, defects of horn and vesicles or focal ulceration at the coronet. Swine vesicular disease lesions can grow out with the horn and may present only as focal defects (Fig. 10.8).

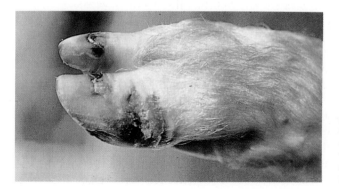

Fig. 10.8
Swine vesicular disease. Chronic focal lesions growing out from the coronary band.

PAIN SENSATION

Pain sensitivity may be increased in irritative or inflammatory disorders or it may be decreased as a result of partial or complete denervation of an area.

Superficial pain is discrete and localized and deep pain is persistent, severe and not readily localized. Superficial pain is tested by pricking with a hypodermic needle but in pigs it is difficult to elicit or recognize a normal response. Increased superficial pain perception (hyperaesthesia) is however the usual means of locating a septic focus or similar focal painful lesion. It therefore plays an essential role in location of most inflammatory musculoskeletal conditions. Deep pain can usually be tested in the pig and is an especially useful procedure in the evaluation of paraplegia. The foot (base of each claw) is pinched with forceps or in adult pigs with hoof testing pliers as necessary to produce the essential vocal or head turning response.

When establishing the response to deep pain it is important to remember that withdrawal of the limb (flexion reflex) is dependent only upon the intact segmental reflex arc and does not provide information on pain sensation, unless accompanied by signs of conscious pain perception. Absence of deep pain response carries an unfavourable prognosis since only severe damage to neural tissue affects the small unmyelinated C fibres which transmit pain impulses. If, in the paraplegic pig, the hindlimb flexion reflex is present but there is bilateral loss of deep pain perception it can be concluded that the peripheral nerve supply is intact and that there is severe damage to the spinal cord.

CONCLUSION

Diagnosis in food animals, unlike diagnosis in companion animals, does not usually require that clinical techniques be pursued in depth since elective post-mortem examinations can be employed to expedite aetiological diagnosis providing that a cost benefit is anticipated. This paper has concentrated on the anatomical localization of lesions in porcine locomotor disorders for it is from such clinical observations that the pathologist can operate most effectively.

When considering differential diagnosis of locomotor diseases of pigs the clinician should always give special consideration to those potential diagnoses which are notifiable diseases. They are for the most part currently exotic disorders of which the clinician may not have had field experience but for which early detection is essential to effective control.

ACKNOWLEDGEMENTS

I thank Dr J. T. Done for helpful criticism and my many other colleagues in the State veterinary service for their interest in providing case material and illustrations.

FURTHER READING

Leman, A. D., Glock, R. D., Mengeling, W. L., Penny, R. H. C., Scholl, E. & Straw, B. (1981). (eds) *Diseases of Swine*, 5th edn. Iowa, Iowa State University Press.

Oliver, J. E. & Lorenz, M. D. (1983). *Handbook of Veterinary Neurologic Diagnosis*. London: W. B. Saunders.

Palmer, A. C. (1976). *Introduction to Animal Neurology*, 2nd edn. Oxford, Blackwell.

Taylor, D. J. (1983). *Pig Diseases*, 3rd edn. Cambridge, Burlington Press.

CHAPTER 11

Lameness in Pigs Associated with Foot and Limb Disorders

BILL SMITH

INTRODUCTION

Lameness is defined by Wells (Chapter 10) as impaired movement or deviation from normal gait. Movement is brought about by functional integration of the nervous system, muscles, tendons, joints, ligaments and the feet. Pain is the most common cause of lameness but any functional disorder of the muscle/skeletal system will also impair or cause abnormal movement.

LAMENESS ASSOCIATED WITH SWOLLEN JOINTS

ARTHRITIS

Cases are usually caused by bacterial infection gaining entry to the joints from the blood stream, (commonly *Streptococcus* species, *Staphylococcus* species, *Corynebacterium pyogenes* and *Escherichia coli*). In pigs, septic polyarthritis (joint ill) is common and usually comes in waves affecting up to 60 % of litters with the percentage of pigs within litters varying from 10 to 100 %. Lameness may appear as early as 4 days of age with swelling of the joints appearing at 7–10 days old. In a few cases (less than 5 %), septic omphalophlebitis (navel ill) may be present but more often than not there is no clinical evidence of the site of entry of infection.

Many pigs will have necrosis of the knees or hock and will also be docked but there is no good evidence to link these lesions with the portal of entry of the organism. The most important routes of entry in the young pig are the tonsils and intestines. However, it is possible that any disruption of the skin or mucous membrane barrier such as bite wounds, badly lacerated gums from faulty teeth cutting or docking and foot lesions might lead to septic arthritis. The causal organism can readily be isolated from early untreated cases.

Mortality may reach 50 % even after treatment and is often related to starvation and overlying. In weaned and finishing pigs septic arthritis can be caused by similar organisms to those involved in neonatal polyarthritis, but *C. pyogenes* is more frequently involved. Cases are always chronic in nature, less susceptible to treatment and always lead to partial or total condemnation at the abattoir. In many cases tail biting or ear biting is a concomitant feature or there may be evidence of healed/old bite wounds.

It has also been suggested that in some cases recrudescence of dormant neonatal infectious arthritis may be the cause. Contaminated needles can also be a source of infection but are more likely to produce a localized abscess. Affected animals may be fevered and arthrocentesis will produce the typical creamy pus. Cases of septic polyarthritis due to *Streptococcus suis II* can present in both weaned and finishing pigs. These are usually secondary to a septicaemia and septic meningitis is also often a sequel.

MYCOPLASMAL ARTHRITIS

Polyarthritis due to *Mycoplasma hyorhinis* occasionally presents as lameness in 3–10-week-old pigs. As the organism is a common inhabitant of the upper respiratory tract stress may precipitate septicaemia and eventually colonization of the synovial membranes as well as other mucous membranes. Animals exhibit mild fever and evidence of peritonitis such as arched-back and tensing of the abdomen. Affected animals may remain lame for up to 6 months. The organism can usually be identified from cultures sown from synovial fluid of early untreated cases (Fig. 11.1). At post-mortem examination, the affected joints contain serosanguineous fluid with fibrin strands while villous hypertrophy is usually obvious. In addition there is often evidence of chronic pleurisy, pericarditis and, or, peritonitis.

Another form of mycoplasmal arthritis which is now more common, is that caused by *M. hyosynoviae* infection. The organism is a common inhabitant of the nasopharyngeal region of young pigs and may gain entry to the joints at an early age without causing disease signs until 12–24 weeks old, usually after the pig has been subjected to some form of stress such as change in management or movement often combined with puberty. There is also evidence to suggest that joint disease associated with *M. hyosynoviae* may be secondary to degenerative joint disease and is often most severe in those joints surrounded by heavy muscle. Affected animals are usually afebrile and reluctant to move or rise. A number of different postures may be adopted depending on the joints affected. When the forelimbs mainly are involved pigs tend to shift weight to their hind legs exhibiting flexion of the carpus, extension of the elbows, tucking of the hindlimbs under the abdomen and curvature of the spine (Fig. 11.2). Whatever the joint involvement the gait is always of a stiff nature and many animals seem "up on their toes". If the carpal or tarsal joints are involved the distension is usually visible and can be palpated but more often the elbow and

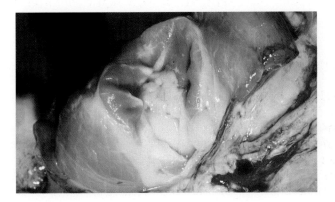

Fig. 11.1
M. hyorhinis infection in the stifle joint. Note excessive serosanguineous fluid and fibrin clot.

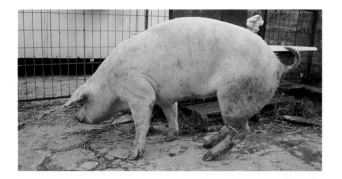

Fig. 11.2
M. hyosynoviae arthritis in a gilt. The weight is shifted on to the back legs, flexing the carpus and extending the elbows. The hindlimbs are tucked under the abdomen and the spine curved.

stifle joints are more severely involved and impossible to detect by palpation. The majority of cases resolve spontaneously in 7–10 days but a number will persist for long enough to require treatment. Post-mortem examination will reveal copious amounts of serosanguineous fluid in the affected joints with attendant villous hypertrophy and hyperaemia of the synovial membrane (Fig. 11.3). There is rarely any involvement of the articular surfaces. Even if suspected, the organism can be difficult to isolate from infected joints. Positive blood titres simply mean that the pig has been exposed to the organism and should not be taken as confirmation of a diagnosis. In short, a non-suppurative acute synovitis without pyrexia in 12–24-week-old pigs is suggestive of *M. hyosynoviae* infection.

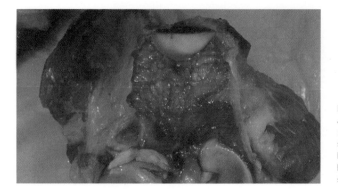

Fig. 11.3
Joint affected by *M. hyosynoviae* arthritis showing villus hypertrophy and hyperaemia of synovial membrane.

GLASSER'S DISEASE

Polyserositis due to *Haemophilus parasuis* (Glasser's disease) is often clinically similar to that caused by *M. hyorhinis* and a similar age group is usually involved. However, when minimal disease pigs or non-immune pigs (up to finishing weight) are introduced to an infected group the disease can often be recognized when cases of meningitis occur while affected animals are more seriously ill, unwilling to move with widespread cyanosis and an oedematous thickening of the ear which is almost pathognomonic (Fig. 11.4). The carpal and tarsal joints are most often affected and are usually swollen and palpably distended. In acute cases a massive septic polyserositis is evident at post mortem (Fig. 11.5) and cultures sown from joints and internal organs will confirm the diagnosis. Arthritis alone is likely to be seen in less than 5 % of cases. It is important to detail all clinical signs and history when submitting selected material to the laboratory as special isolation techniques have to be used for the isolation and identification of the organism.

SWINE ERYSIPELAS

Lameness may accompany the acute/subacute form of the disease which is well recognized by all persons concerned with pig keeping. Affected animals exhibit weight-bearing lameness and more often than not have more than one limb affected. Animals are unwilling to move and usually have an arched-back with hind legs tucked under the abdomen (Fig.

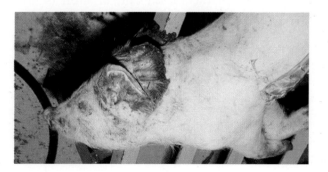

Fig. 11.4
Glasser's disease.

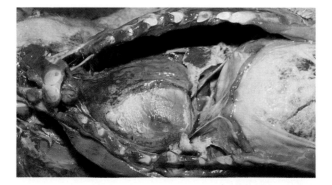

Fig. 11.5
Massive septic
polyserositis seen at
post mortem.

11.6). Diagnosis rarely requires the use of laboratory techniques because of the general clinical signs. In acute cases
affected joints may be swollen and contain serosanguineous
fluid with fibrin strands or flakes of purulent material. In
chronic cases lameness is often the only clinical sign and
diagnosis is not so easy. Cases follow an acute outbreak but
can often appear spontaneously. The progress of the disease
is often slow and insidious. The carpus and tarsus are most
commonly affected and joints gradually become enlarged to
the extent that chronic tenosynovitis may be suspected.
Palpation will reveal a firmness due to fibrosis and periostosis
round the joint. As in other types of weight-bearing lameness
the stance and gait adopted by the animal will depend on the
number of joints affected. At post-mortem examination an
excessive amount of serosanguineous fluid will be noted (Fig.
11.7) along with purulent material and fibrin. The synovial
membranes will exhibit proliferation and hyperaemia. Evidence of exostosis and periarticular fibrosis is almost pathognomonic. In advanced cases ulceration and erosion of the
articular cartilage may be observed. The diagnosis may be
confirmed by positive serology and bacteriology of joint fluid.

SECONDARY INFECTION DUE TO TRAUMA

Young pigs

The introduction of unsuitable perforated floors in farrowing
pens in the past 15 years has caused serious intractable

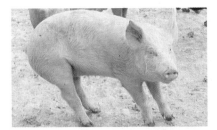

Fig. 11.6
Acute erysipelas in the hock joint.

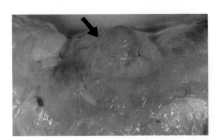

Fig. 11.7
Bulging of synovial membrane (arrow) caused by excessive synovial fluid.

outbreaks of lameness in suckling pigs in some cases. Likewise, erosion of concrete floors exposing a rough/sharp aggregate can cause similar problems. This usually presents as lameness with apparent swelling of the joints between 6 and 10 days of life and is nearly always diagnosed as "joint ill". In fact careful examination of most cases at post mortem will reveal that the majority are suffering from septic tenosynovitis tracking up from the digits which may or may not still have scars of healed erosions. Surprisingly, erosions as seen (Fig. 11.8) seem to cause little apparent lameness and will often have healed completely by 14 days old. Only 3–8 % of erosions lead to infections tracking up the leg. Once swelling around the claws and joints becomes chronic (Fig. 11.9) response to treatment is poor. A mixture of organisms may be involved but streptococci predominate. Control can be achieved by repairing or replacing the floor.

Older pigs

In older pigs the problem is usually apparent as foot rot which is again induced by floor conditions and usually presents as

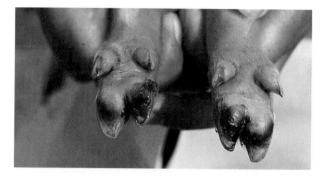

Fig. 11.8
Claws of a 3-day-old
piglet showing
erosion of medial
claws.

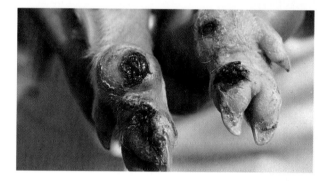

Fig. 11.9
Lower hindlimbs of
an 18-day-old piglet
showing chronic
lesions on heels and
accessory digits.

lameness associated with erosion in either the heel, toe or sole (Fig. 11.10) sometimes in conjunction with whiteline lesions and false sandcracks. Secondary infection from these lesions will often lead to septic laminitis (bush foot) (Fig. 11.11) or to infection tracking up the leg.

LAMENESS WITH NO OBVIOUS SWELLING OF JOINTS

The markedly improved, rapidly growing pig of today is more susceptible to limb and joint disorders which have not yet been clearly differentiated on aetiological or pathological grounds and this can cause real problems for both the practitioner and pig breeder alike.

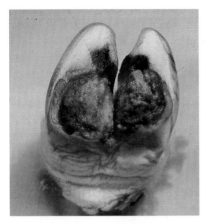

Fig. 11.10
Bilateral erosion of sole of the claw of a bacon pig.

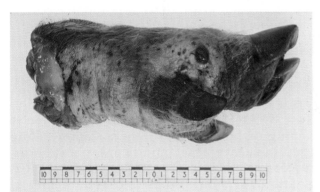

Fig. 11.11
Lower limb bacon
pig showing bush
foot. (Photos courtesy
R. H. C. Penny.)

DEGENERATIVE JOINT DISEASE

This may be the best all-embracing term, which does not imply primary infection, to describe lesions also referred to as osteoarthrosis, osteochondrosis, and osteoarthritis. Osteochondrosis is a fairly specific lesion in the articular/epiphyseal cartilage complex which sometimes leads to cartilaginous lesions (Figs. 11.12 and 11.13) on the articular surface of the joint, producing flaps, craters and "joint mice". Osteochondrosis has been observed in pigs as early as the first week of life without clinical signs and this "normal" condition may persist throughout the pig's life. When clinical signs do occur they usually appear between 4 and 6 months old. These vary tremendously from vague leg weakness to severe lameness depending on which joints are affected and to what extent they are affected. If the articular cartilage remains intact many animals will recover spontaneously. The hip, stifle and elbow joints are most commonly involved and clinically the problem can mimic arthritis due to *M. hyosynoviae*. Rapid growth rate, heavy muscling, lack of exercise, puberty and nutritional status are all factors thought to be involved in precipitating clinical disease from what some consider to be a normal lesion in the young rapidly growing animal. Epiphyseolysis is the name given to separation of the femoral head at the epiphysis which may be bilateral in some cases and usually affects gilts, young boars or newly weaned first litter gilts. The condition causes severe lameness and the prognosis is poor. A dog-sitting position is often assumed as the pig has great difficulty in rising and maintaining stability (Fig. 11.14). Apophyseolysis is separation of the tuber ischii and the same comments apply as for epiphyseolysis.

LAMENESS ASSOCIATED WITH NUTRITION

Rickets is a disease of the rapidly growing young pig and is primarily a softening of bone due to mineralization failure associated with an imbalance of vitamin D and phosphorus. The disorder only occurs after weaning and is now rare. It is characterized by stiffness, unthriftiness and abnormality of gait due to bending of long bones and pain around the joints

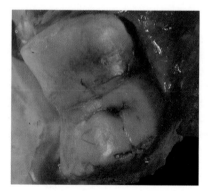

Fig. 11.12
Femoral condyles – note thinning of articular cartilage and fissure.

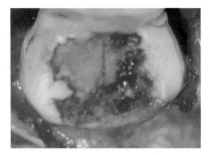

Fig. 11.13
Humoral condyle in a bacon pig showing severe erosion of articular cartilage.

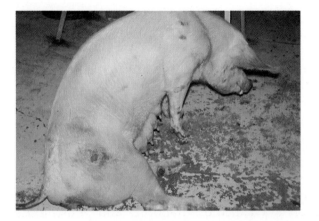

Fig. 11.14
Sow with unilateral epiphyseoysis in the dog-sitting position.

which are occasionally swollen. Osteomalacia is the equivalent of rickets in the adult animal and usually presents as stiffness and acute lameness due to fractures of the limbs or vertebrae. It should be suspected when a 1–3-year-old dam is found recumbent after weaning or service. Osteoporosis results in reduced amount of bone which is itself qualitatively normal, i.e. the ratio of ash to matrix is normal. Diets imbalanced for minerals and composed mainly of cereal are likely to lead to osteoporosis in any age of animals. Fracture of the long bones and vertebra can result. Biotin-responsive lameness has been noted in a number of herds. Animals become lame because of soft claw horn which is more susceptible to erosion and penetration with resultant cracks and secondary infection. Older affected animals may not respond to extra biotin in the diet but the prevalence of lameness in gilts and young sows

Table 11.1 Lameness – foot and limb disorders

Lesion or condition	Infection Primary	Secondary	Joint swelling	Tenosynovitis	Nerve lesions	Bone lesions	Muscle lesions	Nutrition factor	Age (days)	Congenital	Hereditary	Remarks
Joint ill	+	–	+	–	–	–	–	–	2–20	–	–	–
Septic arthritis	–	+	+	+/–	–	tails?	–	–	20–200	–	–	–
M. hyosynoviae	+	–	+	–	–	–	–	–	70–170	–	–	Well muscled
M. hyorhinis	+	–	+	–	–	–	–	–	21–170	–	–	Polyserositis
Glasser's disease	+	–	+	–	–	–	–	–	21–100	–	–	Polyserositis
Erysipelas	+	–	+	+/–	–	+/–	–	–	24–100	–	–	Skin lesions
Neonatal trauma	–	+	+/–	+/–	–	+/–	–	–	4–21	–	–	Floors
Foot rot	–	+	+/–	+/–	–	+/–	–	–	60–170	–	–	Floors
Biotin responsive	–	+	+/–	–	–	–	–	+	180→	–	–	Skin/infertility
Degenerative joint disease	–	–	+/–	–	–	+	–	–	120–200	–	–	Fast growth; well muscled
Epiphyseolysis	–	–	–	–	–	+	–	Ca?	200→	–	–	–
Apophyseolysis	–	–	–	–	–	+	–	Ca?	200→	–	–	–
Rickets	–	–	+/–	–	–	+	–	+	14–70	–	–	–
Osteomalacia	–	–	–	–	–	+	–	–	250→	–	–	–
Osteoporosis	–	–	–	–	–	+	–	–	250→	–	–	–
Teschen/Talfan	+	–	–	–	+	–	–	–	0→	–	–	Paresis
Aujeszky's disease	+	–	–	–	+	–	–	–	0–60	+/–	–	Fits; infertility
Swine fever	+	–	–	–	–	+/–	–	–	0→	+/–	–	Classic signs

Foot-and-mouth	+	–	–	–	–	–	–	3→	–	–	Vesicles
Swine vesicular disease	+	–	–	–	–	–	–	3→	–	–	Vesicles
Congenital tremor	+/–	–	+	–	–	–	–	0–56	+	–/–	Five causes
Adult tremor	–	–	+	–	–	–	–	100–700	+	?	Landrace mainly
Vitamin A (newborn)	–	–	+	+	–	–	+	0–21	+	–	–
Vitamin E deficiency	–	–	+	–	–	–	+	–	–	–	Goose stepping
Vitamin B$_2$	–	–	+	–	–	+	+	2–42	–	–	–
Cu deficiency	–	–	–	–	+	–	+	1–6	–	–	Vitamin E link
Fe toxicity	–	–	+	–	+	–	–	40–70	–	–	–
Se toxicity	–	–	+	–	–	–	–	14–180	–	–	Interaction
Monensin/tiamulin toxicity	–	–	–	–	+	+	–		–	–	
Sunburn	–	–	+	+	–	–	–	7→	–	–	Skin lesions
Organophosphorus poisoning	–	–	+	+	–	–	–	21–180	–	–	21-day gap
Organoarsenic poisoning	–	–	+	–	+	–	–	21–180	–	–	–
Porcine stress syndrome	–	–	–	–	+	–	–	21–180	–	+	–
Back muscle necrosis	–	–	–	+	+	–	–	0–3	–	+/–	Mainly Landrace
Splayleg	–	–	–	+	–	–	–	21–56	–	+	Fatal
Pietrain creeper syndrome	–	–	–	+	–	–	–	0	+	–	Fatal
Thick leg	–	–	–	+	–	–	–	200→	–	?	–
Spondyiitis	–	–	–	–	–	–	–		–	–	–

should drop dramatically following additional inclusion rate if the condition is present in the herd. Lameness due to biotin deficiency may also be suspected when there is a degree of alopecia, dry crusty skin and infertility in the herd.

LEG WEAKNESS

Leg weakness is a description given to a variety of abnormal gaits and locomotion and is not a specific disorder. In all cases the disorder should either be ascribed to very poor conformation or to one or other of the recognized pathological conditions of the joints or bone. Several workers have admitted that osteochondrosis is likely to be present in many cases of so-called leg weakness. If a problem with leg weakness arises a number of affected animals should be culled and subjected to in-depth investigation including gross pathology, X-ray, histological examination and bone analysis so that a more accurate diagnosis can be made. Clinical signs include knock-knee, cross-legs, walking on toes, cow hocked or poor conformation.

CONCLUSION

There are many causes of lameness (see Table 11.1) and several of these are either associated with whole body infections or with specific disorders outwith the limb. Clinicians must take care to examine in detail the history, epidemiology and any unusual presenting features of a problem before proceeding to individual clinical examinations. Indeed some time should be given to observing the behaviour of animals in their natural surroundings. Above all, one should be aware of the advice attributed to Hughling Jackson "The study of things caused must precede the study of causes of things."

Control

CHAPTER 12

Vaccination Programmes for Pigs

MARK WHITE

INTRODUCTION

Many endemic infectious diseases are strongly influenced by the environmental and management conditions prevailing on the modern pig unit. For certain diseases a vaccination programme, undertaken with guidance from a veterinarian, is a useful component of a herd health control programme (Table 12.1).

This review will concentrate on clinical experiences with vaccines that are commercially available in Great Britain. Vaccines can be used as follows:

Table 12.1 Diseases covered by commercial vaccines available in the UK

Erysipelas
Parvovirus
Atrophic rhinitis
Colibacillosis
Clostridial enteritis (*C. welchii* type C)
Clostridium oedematiens (novyi) type B
Salmonella cholerae-suis
Tetanus
Anthrax } (Northern Ireland only)
Aujeszky's disease

(1)   Directly to stimulate and provide active immunity.
(2)   Indirectly to provide passive immunity for the offspring.
(3)   To protect the sow and the litter.

In practice, most vaccination programmes operate in the breeding herd.

ERYSIPELAS

THE DISEASE

Despite the existence for many years of low-cost vaccines for use against erysipelas, the disease is not uncommonly encountered in the field. There are three clinical manifestations:

(1)   Peracute form. As a sudden death mainly in fattening pigs
(2)   Acute form. The classic "diamonds" associated with extreme pyrexia (Fig. 12.1). Reproductive failures (e.g. abortion, return to service and boar infertility) are frequent sequelae.
(3)   Chronic form. Sometimes secondary to acute disease. It is often associated with necrosis of the extremities (tail, ear tips), lameness from joint lesions and valvular endocarditis.

INDICATIONS FOR VACCINATION

All breeding stock including boars should be vaccinated. Fattening pigs should be vaccinated when outbreaks are anticipated or have been known to occur under the prevailing environmental and managemental conditions. The individual dose of all erysipelas vaccines available in the UK for pigs is 2 ml.

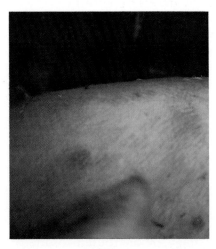

Fig. 12.1
Acute erysipelas in a sow – diamonds.

USE OF VACCINES

The commercially available vaccines in the UK are killed, adjuvented suspensions of *Erysipelothrix rhusiopathiae* and are recommended for subcutaneous use (Table 12.2).

Breeding stock must receive a primary course of two injections – the interval dependent upon the particular vaccine used. Programmes usually start in incoming maiden gilts and boars although *some* vaccines can be given to pregnant animals.

It is important to establish the vaccination status of purchased breeding stock, with dates of each dose administered being provided on delivery. In the recent past, three outbreaks of erysipelas have been seen in pregnant gilts which had been sold fully vaccinated but which, inquiries revealed, had not

Table 12.2 Erysipelas vaccines (all PML)

Vaccine	Manufacturer
Erysorb Plus	Hoechst
Suvaxyn Erysipelas	Duphar
Swine Erysipelas Vaccine	Pitman-Moore
Eryguard	Smith Kline Beecham Animal Health

received two doses of the primary course before delivery; a further outbreak occurred where the interval between the two doses of the primary course was incorrect.

Booster injections are required every 6 months – either on an individual basis, say at weaning, or on a herd basis if the vaccine is safe for use in pregnant animals. In all cases, records of vaccine doses administered to each animal should be kept. Fattening pigs should, where appropriate, be vaccinated in anticipation of disease. A single dose will normally suffice.

DISEASE BREAKDOWN

Confirmed outbreaks of erysipelas infection sometimes occur in vaccinated herds, and can usually be attributed to one or more of the following:

(1) Failure to provide a primary course of vaccination.
(2) Inappropriate interval between the two initial doses.
(3) Excessive environmental challenge associated with poor hygiene.
(4) Stress – including intercurrent disease – particularly at the time of vaccination.
(5) Missed doses, especially in boars.
(6) Poor storage of the vaccine.
(7) Out of date vaccine.
(8) Dirty injection or faulty technique (including vaccines previously contaminated on farm before use) (Fig. 12.2).

In some instances the possibility of strains of the causal organism not being present in the vaccine must be considered.

PARVOVIRUS

In contrast to erysipelas, vaccination against parvovirus infection is relatively new and relatively expensive, but in susceptible populations its use can be cost effective.

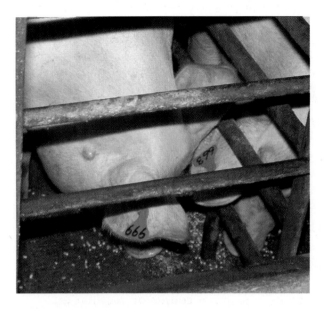

Fig. 12.2
Abscess resulting
from a faulty injection
with erysipelas
vaccine.

THE DISEASE

Infection with parvovirus in the pig may cause disease in the developing embryo and fetus that results in fetal death and either embryo reabsorption or mummification (Fig. 12.3). Thus, the initial signs of a disease outbreak may be a slight increase in returns to service, particularly at irregular intervals, followed by a reduction in litter size and an increase in the incidence of mummified pigs. Occasionally there will be a reduction in piglet birthweight/viability or high stillbirth rate. Abortion caused by parvovirus infection is rare.

INDICATIONS FOR VACCINATION

In view of the highly variable behaviour of the virus within different populations, and the relatively high cost of the vaccine, it has been found that routine blood sampling of a proportion of the female breeding stock (5–10 % at any one time) on a 6–12 monthly basis can be of value in determining the immune status of the herd by measuring haemagglutinating inhibition titres (HI). Sampling over several years has

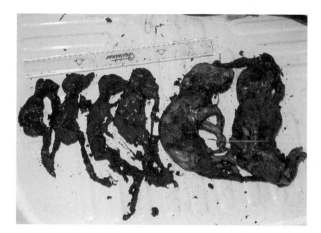

Fig. 12.3
Parvovirus infection in
a susceptible
pregnant sow,
showing progressive
fetal death and
mummification.

revealed a number of different and changing immunity patterns within herds.

The first is a classical cyclical picture of the disease which tends to be seen in smaller herds. In these herds, clinical outbreaks of the disease result in most animals becoming infected and producing high levels of HI antibody. However, as new gilts enter the herd after active virus has subsided, they may not become infected and remain seronegative. As more gilts enter the herd, there is an increase in susceptible animals and as older immune sows leave there is a gradual loss of immunity on a *herd basis*. This leaves a highly susceptible situation ready for re-infection. Regular blood sampling will identify the immune status of the herd.

In large herds parvovirus infection is often endemic. Provided the maiden gilt is exposed to infection as soon as maternal immunity wanes (*this can take up to 7 months or longer*) the herd will remain seropositive. Major outbreaks of disease in existing stable large herds appear to be relatively unusual. Vaccination of such herds appears unnecessary but might be indicated in the gilt because of the variable number of animals seronegative at point of service in spite of attempted exposure to virus.

A third pattern of immunity may be seen in larger herds where integration of the maiden gilts is poor. Here, exposure to parvovirus is only intermittent. In such herds maiden and pregnant gilts may remain seronegative but seroconvert during pregnancy or in later parities where contact with sows is increased. This may also be seen where maiden gilts are served at a young age (i.e. less than 7 months). In these herds, outbreaks of disease can be seen mainly in the younger breeding stock if vaccination is not used. It should be noted that infection will only result in disease in the fetus if it occurs in a susceptible animal during the first 60–70 days of pregnancy.

Where there is a preponderance of young breeding animals in a newly established or restocked unit, or where rapid herd expansion is taking place, immunity to parvovirus is often poor and outbreaks of disease are common. Therefore, in such situations, all gilts should receive one dose of vaccine 2 weeks before service and again 2 weeks after farrowing. In addition, blood sampling of the herd should be carried out 6 months after the first farrowings.

The recommended dose for the commercial vaccines listed (Table 12.3) is 2 ml per sow or gilt.

EFFICACY OF THE VACCINE

The use of commercially available killed vaccines does not produce high HI titres (usually less than 1/40) but titres of less than 1/5 have been shown to be protective.

The introduction of the two oil-based parvovirus vaccines, Suvaxyn Parvo 2 and Porculin has led to claims of extended protection. Any potential advantages of using these vaccines must be weighed against the damage that oil adjuvants can do to the pig (e.g. production of sterile abscesses) and, particularly in the light of COSHH regulations, the potential for serious operator injury should the products be accidentally

Table 12.3 Parvovirus vaccines (POM)

Vaccine	Manufacturer
Pig Parvo Vaccine	Pitman-Moore
Porculin	Pitman-Moore
Suvaxyn Parvo	Duphar
Suvaxyn Parvo 2	Duphar
Nobi-Porvac Parvo	Intervet

self injected. N.B. A number of other vaccines mentioned in this review are similarly oil based.

DISEASE BREAKDOWN

Parvovirus has tended to be used as an excuse for many reproductive failures in the pig. True breakdowns in vaccinated stock have not been seen in this practice where vaccination of identified susceptible groups of animals has been carried out correctly.

When disease appears in vaccinated animals it may be due to:

(1)   Poor vaccination technique, storage or use of the vaccine.
(2)   An inadequate programme of vaccination.
(3)   Gilts vaccinated and served too young.

The data sheet recommends vaccination of boars on a regular basis. Experience has shown that up to 75 % of boars have protective HI titres upon delivery. Furthermore, infection does not produce disease in the boar and the vaccine does not prevent infection. For these reasons, the policy has been not to vaccinate boars in herds under the care of this practice.

ATROPHIC RHINITIS

Atrophic rhinitis (Figs 12.4 and 12.5) is a multifactorial disease which may be associated with infection with *Bordetella bronchiseptica*, *Pasturella multocida* types A, B and D, and inclusion body rhinitis (cytomegalovirus). Environmental conditions, particularly in the farrowing and weaning areas, play a significant part in the initiation of the disease and any control programme must take this fact into account and corrections made accordingly.

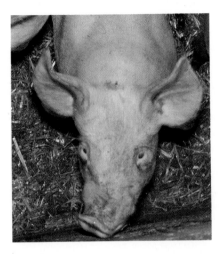

Fig. 12.4
Severe atrophic rhinitis.

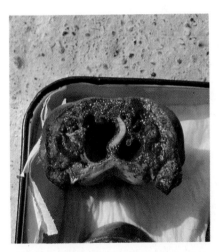

Fig. 12.5
Sectioned snout of a pig severely affected with
atrophic rhinitis.

VACCINES

Table 12.4 lists the commercial vaccines available in the UK
and these all contain *Bordetella* species antigens – either alone
or in combination with some *Pasturella multocida* strains.

Table 12.4 Atrophic rhinitis vaccines (all POM)

Vaccine	Manufacturer	Antigen	Recommended dose	
			Gilts/sows (ml)	Piglets (ml)
Atrovax	Pitman-Moore	B. bronchiseptica	2	1
Delsuvac	Mycofarm	B. bronchiseptica P. multocida type A	2	2
Nobi-Vac ART	Intervet	B. bronchiseptica P. multocida type D (2 strains)	2	Not recommended
Suvaxyn Rhinitis	Duphar	B. bronchiseptica	1	1

USE OF VACCINATION

Use of vaccination to control atrophic rhinitis can be considered in association with environmental correction, medication programmes and managemental changes. Some vaccines are recommended for use in sows or in young pigs but in practice the best results seem to have been obtained by vaccinating the breeding herd and relying on colostral transfer of immunity. Use of vaccination in young pigs is often extremely disappointing.

VACCINATION FAILURE

Use of commercial vaccines can often help in the control of an outbreak of atrophic rhinitis but in the absence of environmental correction results can be extremely disappointing. Likewise, many *apparent* vaccine failures might be due to the presence of toxigenic *P. multocida* type D strains not included in the vaccines. As with other vaccines, correct storage, injection technique and vaccination programme are of paramount importance.

COLIBACILLOSIS

Disease associated with certain pathogenic strains of *Escherichia coli* is very common in the young pig. The most severe disease is seen in the neonatal pig and post-weaned animal, and it is in the former where vaccination has been of the greatest benefit (Fig. 12.6).

USE OF VACCINES

Table 12.5 includes vaccines that contain killed adjuvented antigens of various serotypes of *E. coli*, adhesion factors and labile toxin. All these vaccines are for use by injection and produce mainly an IgG response in serum which is transferred into the colostrum. There is little IgA response and therefore little immunoglobulin raised by the vaccine is present in the milk.

Protection would appear to be required within the lumen of the gut rather than from absorbed antibodies as control of *E. coli* associated enteric disease using these vaccines is often disappointing beyond 4 days of age. However, up to this age they can be highly effective provided that adequate suckling occurs over the critical first 12 h of life. It should always be remembered that scours in piglets more than 1 week old are

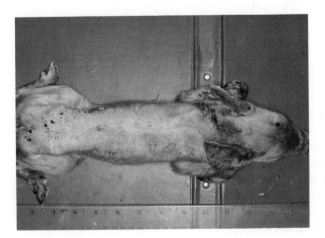

Fig. 12.6
Dehydration and death resulting from neonatal *E. coli* 0149 (Abbotstown strain) infection.

Table 12.5 *E. coli* vaccines (all PML)

Vaccine	Manufacturer	Antigen	Gilt/sow Dose (ml)
Ecopig	Smith Kline	Labile Toxin	5
Gletvax 5	Pitman-Moore	Specific serotypes + K88	5
Nobi-Vac Porcol 5	Intervet	Labile Toxin + K88ab, K88ac, K99 and 987P	2
Porcovac	Hoechst	Specific serotypes	5
Serovax*	Hoechst	Specific serotypes (+ hyperimmune serum)	10
Suvaxyn E. coli P4	Duphar	K88, K99, 987P and F41 Adhesins	2
Intagen	Colborn Dawes	Specific serotypes	1

*Multiple vaccine.

frequently of multiple aetiology (e.g. rotavirus, coccidia, etc.).

The use of an *E. coli* vaccine should be considered where persistent and recurrent disease occurs and is confirmed as being associated with pathogenic *E. coli* strains. It should also be considered for a newly established herd with a preponderance of gilts, and in a breeding herd expansion programme.

Vaccination programmes for breeding stock vary with each commercial vaccine; the data sheet should be consulted for specific recommendations.

FAILURE OF THE VACCINE

Assuming that neonatal disease is associated with pathogenic *E. coli* strains, failure of vaccination procedures may be due to the presence of strains not included in the vaccine; inadequate vaccination programmes or injection techniques; or excessive exposure to infection or poor colostrum intake. As with most control programmes, management must be of a high standard. The standards of hygiene in the farrowing area are very important.

INTAGEN (ORAL VACCINATION)

This involves a complex combined programme incorporating injectable killed adjuvanted *E. coli* antigens combined with infeed antigens. It is used in both for sows, gilts and weaners. The higher costs of such a progamme require careful consideration as to the extent and severity of a problem before its use. The presence of gut (mucosal) stimulation produces mainly an IgA response intended to be protective over the prolonged period of administration. Injection of sows before farrowing, in addition to infeed dosing, stimulates an IgM response – reflected in colustrum – which is said to give better protection to the neonate than IgG stimulated by other vaccines.

CLOSTRIDIAL DISEASE

Severe neonatal enteritis associated with *Clostridium welchii (perfringens)* type C can be a serious disease particularly in extensive systems, although it occurs in highly intensive pig units. Vaccination is indicated in problem herds with recurring disease or in a high-risk situation (Table 12.6).

For the protection of the neonate, a vaccination programme for sows is required which involves a primary course of two doses given subcutaneously at 6 and 2 weeks before farrowing, with boosters 2 weeks prior to farrowing at each subsequent parity. While 2 ml doses often appear adequate, some of the manufacturers recommend that the dose should be higher. In practice, it may be necessary to work up to higher doses if protection is inadequate.

Clostridium oedematiens (novyi) type B infection in sows, producing sudden deaths with "Aero chocolate" livers on post-mortem examination, can similarly be controlled with vaccines. Vaccination should be timed to give maximum protection at the stage in the reproductive cycle when disease is seen (most frequently in late pregnancy).

Tetanus (Fig. 12.7) is seen sporadically in young pigs – most frequently as a result of poor castration technique. While vaccination via sows is feasible it should not be necessary with appropriate attention to management and surgical techniques.

Table 12.6 Clostridial vaccines

Vaccine	Manufacturer	Individual sow dose recommended (ml)	Relevant organisms covered
Covexin 8	Pitman-Moore	up to 5	*C. welchii* C *C. oedematiens* B *(C. tetani)*
Heptavac	Hoechst	up to 5	*C. welchii* C *C. oedematiens* B *(C. tetani)*
Lambivac	Hoechst	up to 2	*C. welchii* C *(C. tetani)*
Quadrivexin	Pitman-Moore	4	*C. welchii* C *(C. tetani)*
Tasvax Gold	Pitman-Moore	up to 4	*C. oedematiens* B *(C. tetani)*
Tasvax 8	Pitman-Moore	up to 4	*C. welchii* C *C. oedematiens* B *(C. tetani)*
Tribovax-T	Pitman-Moore	2	*C. oedematiens* B

N.B. These vaccines are only licensed for use in sheep ± goats ± cattle with the exception of Lambivac which is licensed for pigs.

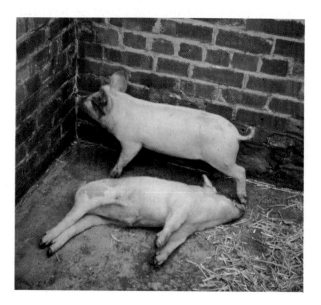

Fig. 12.7
Tetanus in young male pigs showing typical rigid extension of limbs and pricked ears.

SALMONELLA CHOLERAE-SUIS

Salmonella cholerae-suis is now an uncommon disease of growing and fattening pigs which may manifest itself in a range of forms from peracute septicaemia (sudden death) to chronic (necrotic) enteritis. Vaccination is only indicated in the face of disease or in high-risk situations.

A single dose of 1 ml per pig is sufficient using a live vaccine (Suscovax) but with the killed multiple vaccine (Serovax) the dose is variable with age (from 3 to 10 ml) and a double dose with a 10 to 14 day interval is recommended (Table 12.7).

CONCLUSION

This brief review describes the range of vaccines available for use in the pig herd and in all cases the veterinary surgeon must play an integral part in ensuring that the correct vaccine is used in the correct way. The programmes described can only form part of a health control package which at all times must remain cost effective to the pig farmer.

In the vast majority of cases where a complaint concerning a vaccine is made, logical investigation by the practitioner will reveal the reason (Table 12.8); however, if a genuine adverse reaction is seen, then this should be reported to the Medicines Unit of the Central Veterinary Laboratory as well as to the vaccine manufacturer (Table 12.9).

Table 12.7 *Salmonella cholerae-suis* vaccines

Vaccines	Manufacturer	Antigen	Dose
Suscovax	Pitman-Moore (POM)	Live strain 6	1 ml
Serovax*	Hoechst (PML)	Killed strains 2 & 4	up to 10 ml depending on age

*Multiple vaccine.

Table 12.8 Vaccination failure – complaint of failure to protect

Investigate: Is diagnosis of breakdown correct?	No	– Vaccination not relevant
	Yes	– Was the correct vaccine used?
		– Was animal actually vaccinated – primary course (including interval booster)
		– Was route of administration and dosage correct?
		– Was vaccine in date?
		– Was vaccine correct stored, i.e. in a refrigerator?
		– Was vaccine taken from new bottle? (beware part used bottles)
		– Was colostrum intake adequate?
		– Ws animal healthy when vaccinated?
		– Was challenge excessive? (e.g. floor hygiene in scour outbreak)
		– Was sterile needle and syringe used?

Table 12.9 Vaccination failure – complaint of adverse reaction

Has a reaction occurred?

→ Yes → Is it directly associated with vaccination?

→ Yes
- Was vaccine appropriate to that animal? (e.g. pregnant)
- Was route of administration and dose correct?
- Was sterile needle and syringe used?

→ No
- Was technique clean?
- Was new bottle used?

→ No (Has a reaction occurred?)
- Was vaccine correctly stored?
- Was vaccine in date?
- Is it an oil based vaccine?

If answer to all questions is yes, refer to manufacturer and, or, the Central Veterinary Laboratory

ACKNOWLEDGEMENTS

I am most grateful to numerous colleagues who have provided back-up data to clinical experiences enabling this review to be prepared.

CHAPTER 13

Disease Prevention in Pig Herds

ALASTAIR DOUGLAS

INTRODUCTION

Methods of disease prevention in pig herds can be complex but the reason for instituting the measures is usually simple: to reduce disease and increase productivity. It is the herdsman who has to put into action the advice which has been given, so the best way of implementing the measures ought to be discussed with him.

The problems which can arise in pig herds are varied and they might include a departure from the norm. For example, an increase in numbers born dead or suckling pig mortality while numbers of pigs born per sow per year may fall. Such departures from standards may be triggered off by management factors, husbandry factors or infectious diseases.

Action may include strategic medication with drugs at specified times to susceptible pigs. For several diseases advice may need to be a combination of medication and husbandry changes; for example, the occurrence of streptococcal meningitis can be prevented with strategic food medication and an increase in the ventilation rate.

The veterinarian is well placed to help pig farmers in this sphere and as part of a team which may include nutritionists, geneticists and environmentalists his contribution can be valuable. The veterinarian will need a sound knowledge of pig keeping and, if difficulties arise, should be prepared to ask other members of the team to help, or get help from other veterinarians.

HERD FAMILIARIZATION

The practitioner must become familiar with the unit. Herd records will need to be studied so that the performance of the unit can be assessed. The unit should also be visited and walked through with the owner and/or head stockman. The disease history of the herd must be established accurately and in detail.

Using the information obtained from these three actions disease preventive measures can be instituted.

PIG HERD RECORDING

Collecting and recording herd data can be simple. In today's economic climate records are necessary and it is vitally important that they are accurate so that good advice can be given. There are five main reasons for keeping records in pig herds:

(1)   Health, productivity and efficiency can be assessed by the stockman, the manager, the owners and advisers. A comparison with other herds is possible.
(2)   Good areas can be highlighted and encouraged.
(3)   Bad areas can be highlighted for further discussion and investigation.
(4)   The necessity for further pathological examination may be indicated.
(5)   The value of the advice given and the changes carried out can be assessed.

TYPE OF RECORDING SYSTEMS

A minimum number of basic facts need to be written down
(Table 13.1). Analysing these facts can be done either manually
or by a computer. The information produced can relate to the
herd as a whole, individual sows or groups of pigs. For the
busy practitioner simple herd records are quite adequate and
will supply sufficient detail so that they can be used in giving
good veterinary advice.

Individual sow records are not considered in detail in this
article; they usually involve the use of a computer. A computer
permits calculations to be done quickly and easily and the

Table 13.1 Basic facts to be recorded on a monthly basis for use in pig
herd recording

Stock numbers
- (1) Boars
- (2) Sows and served gilts
- (3) Maidens
- (4a) Culls/deaths – sows
- (4b) Culls/deaths – boars

Service area
- (5) Number of 1st services
- (6) Number of 2nd services
- (7) Number of 3rd services

Farrowing area
- (8) Number of farrowings
- (9) Number of pigs born alive
- (10) Number of pigs born dead
- (11) Number of sows weaned
- (12) Number of pigs weaned
- (13) Number of pigs transferred to finishing area
- (14a) Deaths – suckling
- (14b) Deaths – weaning
- (14c) Deaths – finishing

Finishing area
- (13) Number of pigs in
- (15) Number of pigs sold (including number of gilts retained for breeding)

Food (tonnes)
- (16) Amount of sow food used
- (17) Amount of pre-weaning (creep) food used
- (18) Amount of post-weaning food used

retrieval of very detailed information is possible. If farmers wish to join a computer scheme for pig records they should be encouraged to do so because a herd analysis is usually available and this can be used by the veterinarian.

Analysis

Analysing the records of a herd should take no longer than 30 min per herd per month when done by hand providing the data are presented correctly. If a computer is used solely for this analysis with a visual display unit in the office, the time will be reduced considerably.

The concept of "group recording" is a technique which is not often used but which offers a compromise between herd recording and individual sow recording. A group of sows, say 10 in number, is expected to perform to certain standards of production and provided these standards for the group are met there is no need for concern. If the performance of these 10 sows falls below the required standards then action is implemented.

For example, 10 sows could reasonably be expected to wean 95 piglets. Thus if 98 piglets were weaned no action is needed because this is above standard or target levels. If 85 piglets are weaned then prompt action is required because this figure is below target. This concept of group recording is often used in outdoor pig keeping.

A SIMPLE RECORDING SYSTEM

It is most important for any recording system to be simple and easy to understand; the writing must be minimal and events must be recorded as they occur each day. The suggested layout for a breeding and production record is shown in Fig. 13.1. From this the basic facts are reported to the veterinary surgeon each month. This information is then analysed and the herd efficiency parameters as illustrated in Fig. 13.2 are calculated and returned to the farmer. The definitions used in this recording system are those found in *Pig Health. Recording*

Production and Finance – a Producer's Guide.

From the facts presented it is possible to analyse and itemize points which can be used to give advice on a monthly or 6-monthly basis. Targets are discussed and agreed with the herd managers and are rarely changed once agreed. Remarks are made where appropriate each month on the form before it is returned to the farm. Identification of sows with tags, notches or shoulder tattoos is of paramount importance and any recording system fails without this.

A VISIT TO A PIG HERD

The records and the analyses must not be taken in isolation. A visit to the unit on a regular basis is an integral part of the system and should be made fortnightly, monthly, quarterly or as agreed. Muirhead (1980) has described such an advisory visit. In the United Kingdom it is a legal requirement to keep a record of all medication.

These records, the visit and the veterinary history can now be used by the practitioner to formulate some preventive measures.

ROUTINE MEDICATION AND TASKS

Preventive measures fall readily into four groups determined mainly by the age of the animal: the piglet; the weaner and finisher; the adult sow and boar; and the young gilt and the young boar. Some of the measures described are essential for good pig keeping while other measures are possibilities suggested as desirable. Where appropriate, an optimum time for carrying out procedures is given.

Batches, e.g. five or 10 sows, work well for management reasons. The "all in – all out" principle is also a good management tool. All in – all out means that pens are emptied of pigs completely; the pen is then mucked out, thoroughly cleaned and allowed to dry for as long as possible before a new batch of pigs is put into the clean pen. On certain farms it may be possible to follow all in – all out policy in several pens at once or even in a whole building. When thoroughly

Identity of sow	Date last farrowed	Date due to farrow	Farrowing date	Litter no.	Litter card no.	Total piglets	No. alive	No. dead	Boar	Weight at	No. of piglet deaths and cause	Number weaned	No. post weaning deaths and cause	Date weaned	Date of 1st service	Boar	Date of 2nd service	Boar	Date of preg check	Finishing deaths	Remarks

Fig. 13.1 Suggested layout for a breeding and production record chart.

FARM HERD RECORDING

NAME _____ Date _____

LOCAL VETERINARY SURGEON _____

	This mth	3 mths	6 mths		
STOCK DATA No. Boars: No. sows & served gilts: No. Maiden Gilts: No. Prod. Pigs:					
FERTILITY DATA Non Return 1st Srv % : No. Sows Farrowed: Farrowing Rate: Litters/Sow/Year:					
FECUNDITY DATA Total Pigs Born A/D: Born Dead % : Av. Born Alive: Av. Pigs Weaned:					
MORTALITY DATA Sows Culled/Dead: Suck Pig Dead % : Weaner Dead % : Fattener Dead % :					
PRODUCTION DATA Pigs Born/Sow/Year: Pigs Weaned/Sow/Year: Pigs Sold/Sow/Year: Tn Sow Food/Sow/Year:					
FEED EFFICIENCY DATA Total Sales: Herd FCR: ADG Weaners gms ADG Finishers gms					

Topical Tip:

Signed:

Fig. 13.2 Example of form to be returned to farmer by veterinary surgeon.

cleaning pig pens remember that dryness and time are very good killers of microorganisms.

PIGLETS

Essential disease preventive measures

(1) Clip teeth to prevent udder soreness as soon as possible after farrowing. Clipping also reduces incidence of facial necrosis of piglets.
(2) Iron supplementation; injections are recommended at

under 7 days old with a dose of 100 mg per piglet. Iron can be given orally during the first 24 h or as a powder on the floor. It can also be given as a dietary supplement for sows at the rate of 250 g extra chelated iron per tonne of sow feed or as hydrated ferrous sulphate at 10 kg/t. This relies on piglets eating sows' faeces.

(3)   Cross fostering evens up litters for size and numbers and is best done under 3 days of age. The author's experience is that it is best to move the big strong piglets. Try to avoid having more than 10 piglets suckling one sow; this might mean weaning piglets from a sow a little early so that she can be used as a nurse sow for extra piglets.

(4)   Water for piglets should be clean, fresh and always available.

(5)   Creep food for piglets is not absolutely necessary when weaning takes place under 3 weeks of age but it is essential when weaning takes place over this age.

(6)   Most piglets are weaned on Thursdays; this avoids weekend work for matings and for most farrowings.

Possible preventive measures

(1)   Dressing the navel with a coloured antibiotic aerosol reduces joint-ill and is best done as soon as possible after birth. The use of jars and teat-dipping cups should be avoided.

(2)   Castration can be done between 1 and 18 days. Some abattoirs accept entire males which have not been castrated.

(3)   Tail docking with blunt scissors or burdizzo (crushing action) is best done on day 1.

(4)   Ear notching or tattooing are best done before day 7. Remember to notch those pigs which have been fostered.

(5)   Antibiotic injections are sometimes given between 1 and 3 days of age for a variety of reasons. On occasions the injection is given in anticipation of a disease; scouring, atrophic rhinitis, joint-ill and streptococcal meningitis are commonly treated this way.

(6)   Vaccination and antiserum injections are occasionally given at about 10 days of age against *Escherichia coli* or clostridial infections.

WEANERS AND FINISHERS

Essential disease preventive measures

(1)   The feed being used should be an appropriate one. The miller will need to be consulted.

(2)   Water should be freely available, with one drinking point to every 10 pigs (Fig. 13.3). Arato drinkers are good.

(3)   A growth promoter will be beneficial on most farms. In addition, copper may be supplemented at a rate of 175 ppm until 60 kg and at 125 ppm thereafter.

(4)   All in – all out management as mentioned above is very worthwhile and can prevent diseases becoming endemic.

Possible preventive measures

(1)   Vitamin E may be injected to prevent mulberry heart disease and hepatosis dietetica. In addition injectable antibiotics against atrophic rhinitis or post-weaning diarrhoea syndrome, and vaccines against atrophic rhinitis (using a bordetella/pasturella vaccine), salmonella or *E. coli* can be given. If an outbreak of disease has occurred make sure the implicated serotypes are included.

(2)   Vitamins and antibiotics may be administered in the drinking water. Electrolytes are commonly given; recent work

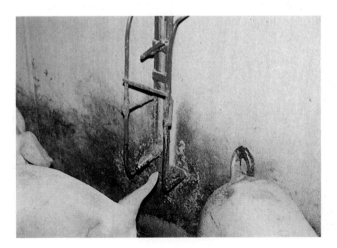

Fig. 13.3
Protected drinker for weaners.

has indicated a need to offer electrolytes to every batch of weaners.

(3)   Vitamins may also be given in the feed, as may antibiotics given for 4–8 weeks or longer after weaning for post-weaning diarrhoea syndrome, bowel oedema, *E. coli* infection, fading weaners and atrophic rhinitis. Infeed anthelmintics are sometimes used and an infeed *E. coli* vaccine is available.

(4)   Bird proofing of pens would be desirable for this age group.

ADULT SOWS

Essential disease preventive measures

(1)   Move adult sows to farrowing accommodation 3–7 days before the expected date of parturition.

(2)   Deworm with a broad spectrum anthelmintic; this is best done on entry to the farrowing crate. Use the cheapest and change it annually. Some hysterectomy-derived herds do not need deworming.

(3)   Wash the udders with warm soapy water to remove sticky ascarid eggs and also other unwanted material like faeces, bedding and dust from food and floor.

(4)   Treat pigs for lice and mange (Fig. 13.4) with a spray, a pour-on or by injection; this is best done on entry to the farrowing house. Some hysterectomy-derived herds do not require this to be done.

(5)   Vaccinate sows against swine erysipelas (*Erysipelothrix rhusiopathiae*) 1–3 days after farrowing.

(6)   Clean water must be freely available. Some work recommends a flow rate of 1.5 l/min; this is quite fast, but does allow the sow to take its fill of water easily. Bite drinkers are probably the best means of supply and reduce wastage (Fig. 13.5).

Possible disease preventive measures

(1)   Dung dosing and the feeding of farrowing house waste to sows in late pregnancy (28–14 days before farrowing) can immunize sows against *E. coli*, (porcine parvovirus and

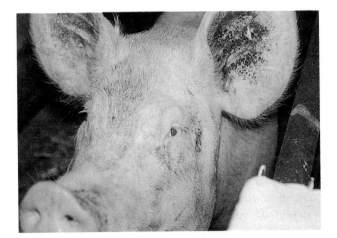

Fig. 13.4
Crusty ear mange in a sow.

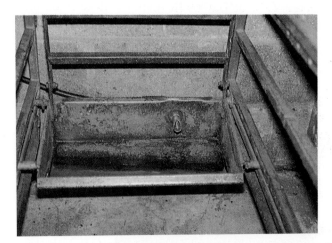

Fig. 13.5
Good position for water point in farrowing house.

transmissible gastroenteritis in the event of an outbreak) and other diseases. In the author's experience it is very hard to abort a sow in late pregnancy so dung dosing can be carried out with confidence and it is strongly recommended. Do not expose sows in early pregnancy to this technique. In the United Kingdom a licence is required from the Ministry of Agriculture if the waste contains animal protein, e.g. fetal membranes or dead and mummified piglets.

(2) Prostaglandins are very useful to induce farrowing. They

should be administered 24 h in advance of the desired time of farrowing. Oxytocin can be given 24 h after prostaglandin if farrowing has not commenced.

(3)   Oxytocin is used on some farms on every sow that has started farrowing. Giving 0.5 ml every half hour is preferable to 2 ml in one dose.

(4)   Injections of vitamin E can be given; this vitamin may be lacking in the progeny at weaning, especially in highly productive sows (e.g. sows which farrow 28 piglets per year).

(5)   Oestrus induction may be carried out in recalcitrant sows (often first litter sows) using a mixture of serum gonadotrophins and human chorionic gonadotrophins. It is rare for every sow to be treated at weaning.

(6)   Sows are vaccinated in mid or late pregnancy against a variety of diseases including atrophic rhinitis, anthrax, clostridia and *E. coli* with manufactured vaccines or antogenous vaccines. Porcine parvovirus vaccine can be given to non-gravid sows. See Figs 13.6 and 13.7 for positions for injecting sows.

BOARS

Possible disease preventive measures

(1)   Swine erysipelas and porcine parvovirus vaccination are essential.

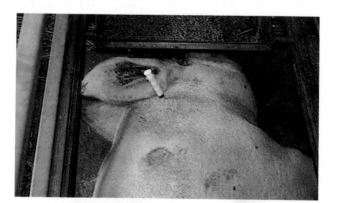

Fig. 13.6
Position for injecting
a sow
intramuscularly.

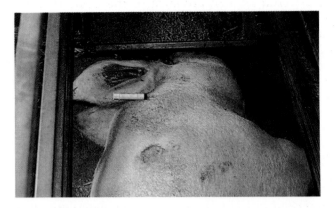

Fig. 13.7
Position for injecting
a sow
subcutaneously.

(2) Dressing for lice and mange control is desirable.
(3) Boars should be dewormed regularly.
(4) Do not forget the boar; he is an important member of the herd.

GILTS AND YOUNG BOARS

Essential disease preventive measures

New purchases must be quarantined for 4 weeks which includes 2 weeks of complete isolation and 2 weeks of integration. This is followed by 2 weeks in the service area before being mated on the third heat (gilts). Home-bred gilts and boars should be taken through the process from integration onwards.

Integration means exposing, in the quarantine station, young gilts and boars to the bacterial and viral populations of the herd. This is done by dung dosing as already mentioned for adult sows or by a cull sow or a convalescent finishing pig being in the same pen or next-door pen if naso-nasal contact is possible.

Vaccination against swine erysipelas, porcine parvovirus, *E. coli* and other diseases can be commenced here. A primary course of two injections may be necessary. Deworming, dressing for lice and mange and also anti-swine dysentery medication can be done in this 2-week integration period.

Vasectomized boars are useful for identifying gilts in oestrus and for giving mating practice to gilts.

COSTS OF A DISEASE PREVENTION PROGRAMME

The cost of advice is usually calculated on the current hourly rate; drugs and medicines and charges for visits are extra. The approximate cost of various medications on a per dose basis as used in a practice in Suffolk is illustrated in Table 13.2.

SUMMARY

A simple recording system which can be used in any veterinary office has been described. The results of the analyses are used when making a visit and to institute disease control measures. Many disease preventive measures essential to pig keeping are discussed. The busy practitioner with just a few pigs under his or her care will need to be familiar with these.

Table 13.2 Approximate cost of some disease control procedures in a Suffolk practice

Treatment	Approximate cost per dose in 1991 (p)
Antibiotics per sow	254
per piglet	25
Electrolyte per 5 l	95
Infeed antibiotics per weaner per day	3
Hormones for treatment of anoestrus	472
Iron injection	8
Lice and mange wash	30
Oxytocin	65
Prostaglandin	200
Vaccines	
Anthrax	70
Atrophic rhinitis	104
Clostridium species	20
Porcine parvovirus	362
Swine erysipelas	21
Vitamin E	43
Water-soluble antibiotics per weaner	7
Wormer and mange injection per sow	207
Oral wormer per sow	100

REFERENCES

Muirhead, M. R. (1980). *Veterinary Record* **106,** 170.
Pig Health. Recording Production and Finance – A Producer's Guide. Produced in association with the Pig Veterinary Society, c/o BVA, 7 Mansfield St, London W1M 0AT.

FURTHER READING

English, P., Smith, W. & Maclean, A. *The Sow – Improving Her Efficiency.* Ipswich: Farming Press.
Taylor, D. J. (1989). *Pig Diseases,* 5th edn. Cambridge, Burlington Press.
Whittemore, C. T. (1980). *Pig Production: The Scientific and Practical Principles.* London: Longman.
Pig Yearbook 1991. Bletchley, Milton Keynes, Meat and Livestock Commission.
Pig Farming. Ipswich, Farming Press.
Pig Veterinary Society Proceedings, obtainable from T. W. Heard, Grove House, Corston, Malmesbury, Wiltshire.
Pig News and Information. Wallingford, CAB.
Leman, A. D. *Diseases of Swine,* 6th edn. Iowa, Iowa State University Press.

Index